Your Complete Guide to Nutrition for Weight Loss Surgery

Sally Johnston

Accredited Practising Dietitian | Accredited Nutritionist

First published in 2013 by Sally Johnston.

Second edition published 2014. Reprinted 2015.

Third edition published 2016.

Design: Regan Birrell and Jayne Freeman.

Food Styling: Rob Paglia, Mel Haynes, Sally Johnston, Robyn McKean.

Photography: Daniel Trimboli.

Some images courtesy of istock.

Edited by Robyn McKean, Judy and Alastair Johnston, Catherine Jarman.

National Library of Australia Cataloguing-in-Publication entry.

Author: Johnston, Sally, author.

Title: Your complete guide to nutrition for weight loss surgery / Sally Johnston.

Edition: Third edition.

ISBN: 978-0-9924346-3-2

Subjects: Obesity--Surgery.

Nutrition.

Reducing diets--Recipes.

Gastrointestinal system--Surgery.

Dewey Number: 617.43

Disclaimers

Medical disclaimer

The information in this book is intended for use as a general reference. It is provided on the understanding that it is intended to motivate and educate but is not a replacement for professional advice. It does not constitute advice of a health care professional on any specific health issue/condition. For specific dietary advice tailored to your individual needs consult an Accredited Practising Dietitian. For advice specific to weight loss surgery, consult a member of the Obesity Surgery Society of Australia & New Zealand (OSSANZ). Accredited Practising Dietitians who are members of OSSANZ are listed on the OSSANZ website: www.ossanz.com.au. The author accepts no responsibility for any failure to seek or follow the advice of a healthcare professional and will not be liable for such failure.

Every effort has been made to incorporate correct information and attribute copyright. No responsibility is taken for errors or omissions.

Use of Commercial Products

It should be noted that this book originated in Australia, hence all commercial products used are available in Australia. In countries other than Australia a dietitian should be consulted regarding the most appropriate products.

At the time of writing, Optifast VLCD®, KicStart® VLCD and Dr. MacLeod's® are the best available products of their type. They are recommended by dietitians and surgeons in the weight loss surgery field in Australia.

Similarly, Benefiber® is considered the best available fibre supplement for this purpose.

Protein supplements based on whey protein isolate are considered superior to the other commercially available forms of protein supplement and are therefore recommended. Chobani® yoghurts and The Complete Dairy™ milk are recommended as at the time of printing, these products had the highest protein content for products of their type. The author has no financial interest in the companies that manufacture or distribute any of these products and has received no incentives to recommend them. BODIE'z clear protein water products are recommend as they are unique products on the Australian market and for this reason, the author is an ambassador for these products.

It cannot be guaranteed that these products will always be the best available as new lines are developed and introduced to the market. The choice of such items should always be discussed with your dietitian.

Contents

Foreword

Good health and great food - this is something everybody wants. But the quest for good health is unfortunately all too commonly taken over by dieting; a predominantly commercial enterprise, which promises much, but rarely delivers. The enjoyment of good food then becomes a distant memory for many people. Sally Johnston's book is as refreshing as it is original, and it rejoices in its ability to provide good food to those who are planning a long-term commitment to their own health. This book, replete with beautiful colour photography and succinct recipes, would not look out of place on a coffee table. But delve deeper and it becomes apparent the degree of detail and wealth of research that has gone into making the dishes a foundation for healthy eating. I can truly say that this volume has been a labour of love for Sally and this more than anything, shines through. Sally Johnston is impeccably credentialed and widely experienced, and I have complete trust in the advice she can deliver. Enjoy this book, enjoy your health and bon appétit!

Justin Bessell

General and Upper Gastrointestinal Surgeon

www.adelaideobesitysurgery.com.au

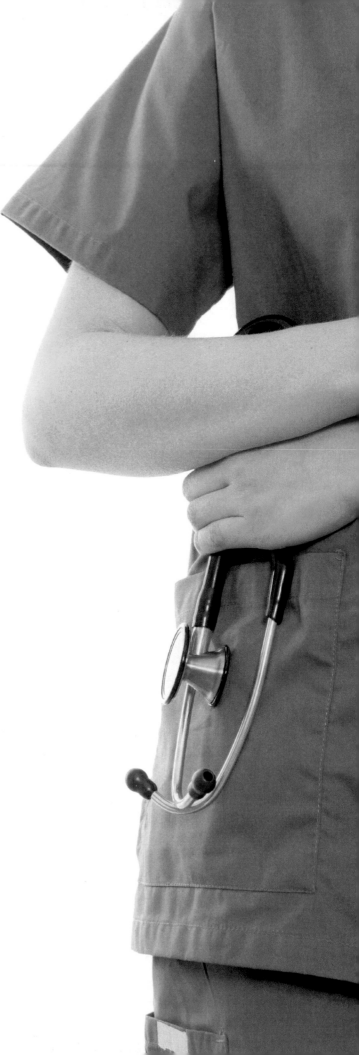

About the Author

Sally Johnston
Accredited Practising Dietitian, Accredited Nutritionist

The founder of *Nutrition for Weight Loss Surgery*, Sally has a Bachelor of Applied Science (Human Movement) and a Master of Nutrition and Dietetics. Sally is an Accredited Practising Dietitian (APD) and Accredited Nutritionist (AN) of the Dietitians Association of Australia (DAA).

Sally has specialised dietetic counselling skills in the dietary management of those undergoing weight loss surgery, having provided dietetic consultations to individuals as part of an holistic, multidisciplinary obesity management team since 2005.

Sally is a regular user of social media to provide a credible source of nutrition information and support for those undergoing weight loss surgery.

Feel free to connect with Sally and share your experiences:

f **facebook.com/nutritionforwls**

W **www.nfwls.com**

e **sally@nfwls.com**

Acknowledgements

- Justine Hawke, Accredited Pratising Dietitian, Accredited Nutritionist and the other half of Nutrition for Weight Loss Surgery
- Catherine Jarman, Accredited Pratising Dietitian, Accredited Nutritionist
- Sharon Dredge, Passionate cook with a gastric band
- Rob Paglia, Chef
- Mel Haynes, Chef
- Daniel Trimboli, Photographer
- Regan Birrell, Graphic Designer
- Jayne Freeman, Graphic Designer
- Robyn McKean, Judy and Alastair Johnston and Catherine Jarman for proof reading and editing
- The team at Adelaide Obesity Surgery for their ongoing enthusiasm and support for my projects
- Leon Cohen and the team at Mercy Bariatrics for sharing their data and experiences regarding sleeve gastrectomy
- Kylie Hearnden for sharing her recipes
- Merril Bohn and Nazy Zarshenas for sharing their wealth of experience in bariatric nutrition
- My many patients from whom I have learned much of what is shared in this book.

At Nutrition for Weight Loss Surgery we offer a whole range of weight loss surgery specific tools, products and support options.

Be sure to check us out at *www.nfwls.com*.

Welcome to the Journey

My first book, *Knife, Fork and Band,* evolved from years of patients asking if there were suitable recipe books for those having gastric band surgery. The response to this book was excellent from both patients and health professionals, hence the decision to expand the book to include all forms of weight loss surgery.

So the *Complete Guide* was born. It combines appetising, healthy and simple recipes, the knowledge of an experienced dietitian, input from a wide range of colleagues in the industry, and many, many lessons learned from weight loss surgery patients over the years.

This book has two components, the 'theory' aspects of weight loss surgery and the recipes.

To help you gain a better understanding of weight loss surgery the *Complete Guide* is broken into the following sections:

- *Gastric Band, Sleeve Gastrectomy and Roux-en-Y gastric bypass surgeries*, as it is important to have a basic understanding of the surgery you have had, or are having, how it works and how it needs to be managed. Each surgery has its own unique aspects that you need to understand for long-term success.
- *Preparing for Surgery and Recovering from Surgery* to ensure the safest possible preparation and outcome, with recipes to help you practically at this time.
- *Food Fundamentals Following Weight Loss Surgery* explores the eating techniques, habits and food choices to ensure a varied and nutritious diet that promotes weight loss and maintaining that weight loss. This section is completed with a range of healthy, yet tasty recipes, which can be used long term to promote good health.
- *Troubleshooting and Common Complaints* deals with some of the potential hiccups you may encounter along your journey.
- *Nutritional Impacts of Weight Loss Surgery and Supplementation* describes the common nutrient deficiencies that can occur following weight loss surgery and the nutrition supplements recommended for each surgery type.

Whilst it is good to have a basic understanding of the theory behind nutrition and weight loss surgery, you will get most enjoyment from the tasty recipes throughout the book. Rigorous nutrition analysis has been undertaken in the development of all recipes; however the result is an easy to read publication for people who have had, or are planning to have weight loss surgery.

To complement the nutrition know-how, a trained diet cook who has been through the dietary stages of weight loss surgery herself has reviewed the recipes. Her expertise on improving flavour, increasing fibre and protein, recipe variations and ensuring the methods were clear and easy to follow was invaluable. Volunteers who have had various forms of weight loss surgery were also involved in 'road testing' the recipes. Their feedback is also incorporated and their comments included.

The recipes are not only for those who have had weight loss surgery, but are generally acceptable for family and friends. Suggestions to modify serve sizes for those who have not had surgery are included.

I hope you find *Your Complete Guide to Nutrition for Weight Loss Surgery* a valuable tool on your weight loss surgery journey.

Sally Johnston

Surgery Types

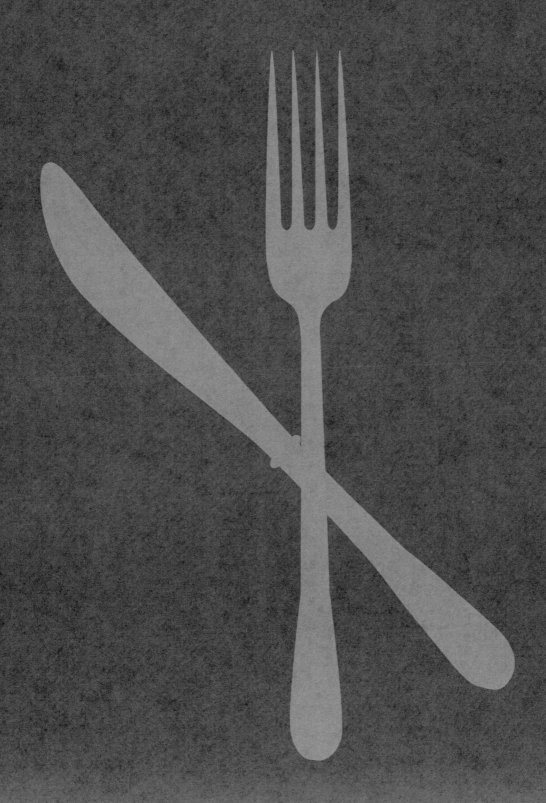

Weight Loss Surgery

The aim of weight loss (or bariatric) surgery is to allow you to feel satisfied after eating a small amount of food. This allows you to eat less food without feeling hungry, allowing a reduction in food intake to promote weight loss. There are various forms of weight loss surgery, as indicated in the diagram. Each form of surgery will be discussed in detail later.

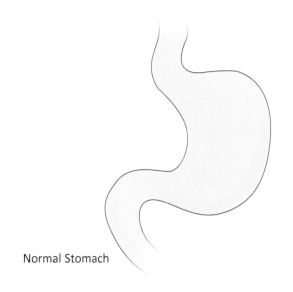

Normal Stomach

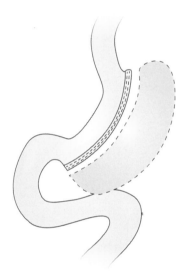

Sleeve Gastrectomy

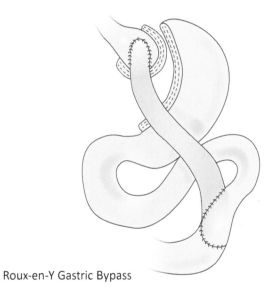

Roux-en-Y Gastric Bypass

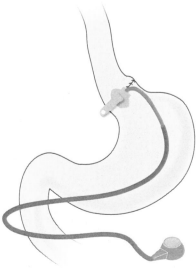

Adjustable Gastric Band

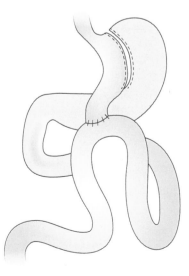

One Anastomosis Gastric Bypass

A Successful Journey

Whilst technically different, what is common to all forms of weight loss surgery is that the surgery itself is just one part of the picture of weight management. Surgery alone does not guarantee you will lose weight; it is a tool that can assist you to lose weight when teamed with lifestyle change.

Colleen Cook is a successful weight loss surgery patient from 1995 and is the author of the best selling weight loss surgery book, *The Success Habits of Weight Loss Surgery Patients*. It is based on her research of the most successful long-term patients and the habits they have in common as they maintain their weight over time. Colleen is also the President of Bariatric Support Centers International, a company that specialises in providing education and support services for those who have had weight loss surgery and the professionals who work with them. Following is a comment from Colleen:

> "Successful patients took personal responsibility for staying in control. They were found to have a general feeling that maintaining their weight was indeed their own responsibility and that surgery was a tool that they used to reach and maintain a healthy weight."

Colleen's words illustrate perfectly that weight loss surgery itself does not cause weight loss. Those undergoing weight loss surgery will need to take responsibility for their lifestyle choices. To achieve the best weight loss results and maintain that weight loss in the long term, you will need to choose healthy and nutritious foods, increase physical activity and maintain regular follow up with your support team.

This book is your partner in ensuring a safe preparation and recovery from surgery and developing a healthy lifestyle for long-term success.

> "It is a great journey."
> - Dana, gastric band -

> "I am more fit now than at any other time in my life."
> - Linda, gastric bypass -

> "It's been life changing, the best thing I have ever done."
> -Beth, gastric band -

> "You need to do the work - it is not a miracle cure."
> - Kristi, gastric band -

> "This surgery has changed my life."
> - Robyn, sleeve gastrectomy -

> "It's changed my whole life!"
> - Frances, gastric bypass -

> "Bariatric surgery is like the cherry on top of the cake, or the tip of a pyramid. It is underpinned by the lifestyle foundations which are a prerequisite to long term success."
> - Dr Justin Bessell, Surgeon -

> "I have chosen to live a better life and although surgery is a drastic measure, I would do it again in a heartbeat."
> - Nina, sleeve gastrectomy -

> "It's extremely helpful to have others walk beside you but no-one else can DO it for you."
> - Judi, gastric bypass -

> "Choosing to have surgery is a big decision and one that will change your way of life as well as the quality of life forever. Be prepared to make the changes required."
> - Dana, gastric band -

Gastric Band Surgery

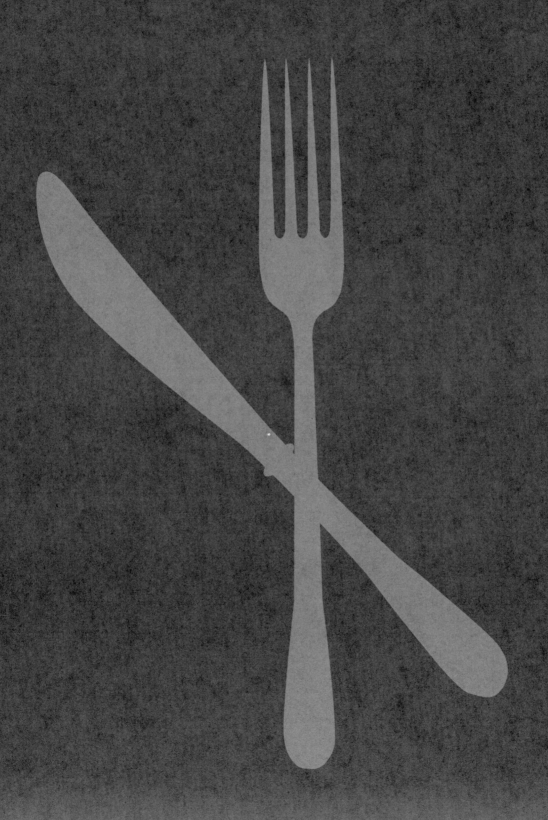

Gastric Band Surgery

How does gastric band surgery work?

A gastric band is a silicone device placed around the upper part of the stomach. It was once believed that the gastric band created a new, smaller stomach above the band, where food would sit before passing into the lower, larger stomach. More recent studies at the Centre for Obesity Research and Education (CORE) in Melbourne have shown this to be incorrect.

The gastric band actually creates a 'funnel' into the larger stomach and exerts pressure on the stomach. Adjusting the gastric band can vary this pressure. The band has an access point called a port, which is stitched to your abdominal muscle deep under the skin. You can usually tell where the port may be as it is likely to sit somewhere under your biggest scar. Your surgeon or bariatric GP uses the port to adjust your gastric band and vary the pressure it places on the stomach. They can inject or remove saline (a salty water) solution via the port to make your band tighter or looser.

When food is eaten our oesophagus, or food pipe, squeezes bites of food down towards the band. Once food reaches the band, contractions of the oesophagus, called peristalsis, will squeeze well-chewed food past the band. In a person with a well-adjusted band, it can take between two to six squeezes of the oesophagus to get a bite of food across the band. One study suggests this process takes at least a minute.

There are nerves in the stomach that detect when our stomach is stretching, and send a message to our brain that we have had enough to eat. One particular nerve involved in controlling our stomach is called the vagus nerve. With a gastric band sitting around the stomach this squeezes the vagus nerve all the time, and more so when you are eating.

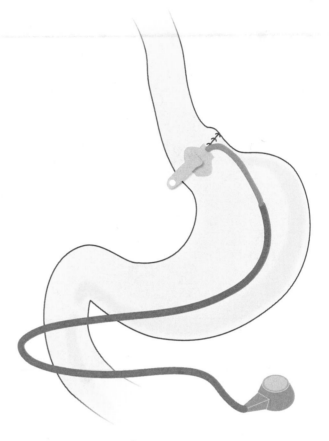

Adjustable Gastric Band

The squeezing process triggers a signal to the brain that you are satisfied, or no longer hungry. This means you feel satisfied on a smaller amount of food than you would have prior to surgery. The constant pressure of the band on the stomach also helps you to feel satisfied for a longer period of time, reducing hunger throughout the day.

Feeling satisfied is different to feeling 'full'. Feeling 'full' means you have eaten to excess. It may indicate food is sitting above the band, either due to eating too quickly, eating large pieces of food or not chewing food well enough. Try to stop eating when you feel satisfied or no longer hungry, rather than full. As bariatric GP Teresa Girolamo says, "It's not about seeing how much you can eat and get away with, it's about seeing how little you can eat to feel satisfied."

Each bite of food must be small and well chewed. An

empty, or uninflated band has an opening the size of a twenty-cent piece. A fully inflated band has an opening the size of a five-cent piece. Most people will have their band adjusted somewhere between the two sizes. If you cut food into the size of a five-cent piece size and chew it well, it is more likely to pass comfortably through the band.

Eating slowly also helps you to eat comfortably. In theory, you should aim to wait a minute between each mouthful of food, however it is not practical to time every mouthful. It is practical to put your cutlery down between mouthfuls and wait until you have swallowed before cutting the next piece of food ready to eat. People with a gastric band who eat quickly, describe a feeling of discomfort in their oesophagus, like a 'traffic jam'. Eating slowly will help avoid this.

Recovering from surgery

When the band is placed, some stomach tissue is wrapped over the band and stitched to hold the band in place, as shown in the diagram. This stitching causes some swelling of the upper stomach making the opening for food or fluid very small. To allow this swelling to subside and the stitches to heal, you must follow a particular recovery diet in the early weeks after surgery. See the *Recovering from Surgery* section (page 52) for more details.

Maintenance

The digestive system remains unchanged after gastric band surgery, hence the risk of nutrient deficiencies is lower than with other surgery types. As you eat less after gastric band surgery, making the most of your food choices will help you obtain all the nutrients required for good health. Preventing nutrient deficiencies is discussed in detail in the *Nutritional Impacts of Weight Loss Surgery and Supplementation* chapter (page 232).

Studies have found that those who had regular follow up after weight loss surgery achieved better weight loss, health improvement, quality of life and food tolerance, than those who did not. Your support team is there to guide you to get the best results following surgery, so make the most of the team and keep in touch! They have all sorts of hints and tips to help you achieve success on your weight loss journey.

Adjusting the Gastric Band

A gastric band adjustment should not be done by your normal GP unless they have had special training. Band adjustments should be done by your surgeon or bariatric GP.

When a gastric band is placed it does not magically cure you of hunger. Some people may experience this, but most will need the band adjusted to feel satisfied on small amounts of food.

The goal of adjusting a gastric band is for you to be in the 'green zone' as indicated in the following diagram. In the green zone you feel satisfied (no longer hungry) on small serves of food and feel satisfied for a longer period of time than you normally would after eating that amount of food. This should therefore assist you to lose weight or maintain the weight lost. The amount of fluid needed to achieve the green zone will differ for each person. Therefore, the number of inflations or fills required or how much fluid you have in your band cannot be compared to others.

Some people believe a tighter band will result in faster weight loss. This is incorrect. As the diagram indicates, a band that is too tight causes poor eating behaviour and unpleasant side effects. An important part of being in the green zone is that you can comfortably eat a good range of solid food. A tight band often means you start to rely on soft, sloppy or liquid foods and this does not help you achieve and maintain your desired weight.

If a gastric band is tight for an extended time it can lead to medical complications. As well as more regular regurgitation, a tight band can put too much pressure on the oesophagus and the stomach, therefore affecting their normal function. Some of the side effects can be quite serious and not reversible. These will generally need to be treated with further surgery.

Getting into the green zone

Has your weight loss stopped even though you are careful to eat well and exercise regularly? Are you putting on some of the weight you had lost?

Are you:

- Eating meals much larger than a bread and butter plate?
- Finding the serve size that used to satisfy you no longer satisfies you?
- Always feeling hungry?
- Snacking all the time?

If you are experiencing any or all of the above, you may need fluid added to your band – this is called an 'inflation' or 'fill'.

Are you:

- Eating sloppy or mushy food because you cannot tolerate solid foods?
- Vomiting regularly?
- Having regular heartburn or reflux?
- Drinking with food to make it easier to eat?

You may need fluid removed from your band – called a 'deflation' or 'de-fill'.

> **"Tighter is NOT better."**
> *- Dr Helen Patroney, Bariatric GP -*

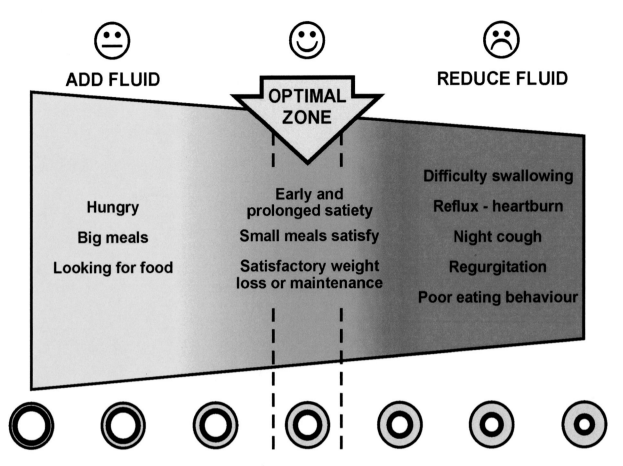

ADD FLUID

OPTIMAL ZONE

REDUCE FLUID

Hungry

Big meals

Looking for food

Early and prolonged satiety

Small meals satisfy

Satisfactory weight loss or maintenance

Difficulty swallowing

Reflux - heartburn

Night cough

Regurgitation

Poor eating behaviour

Courtesy of Centre for Obesity Research and Education, Monash University.

After band adjustments

After your band is adjusted you should make sure it feels comfortable before you leave the clinic. Always have a drink of water to make sure the band is not too tight. If the water does not move through your band, don't leave before speaking to your doctor.

After a band adjustment, take extra care to eat slowly and chew well. Sometimes an adjustment will cause some swelling making it more difficult to eat. Some people find it is best to return to a soft diet following an inflation to allow any swelling to settle. However, if you need to stay on a soft diet longer than a couple of days, call your surgeon or bariatric GP. You must be able to eat healthy, solid food to be using your band to its best effect.

If you find that the inflation has not changed the amount you can eat, you may need a further adjustment/adjustments to get you into the green zone.

Eating and Drinking with a Gastric Band

How much should I be eating?

To understand how much food you should be eating, it is important to understand how the band works. The band does not create a new, smaller stomach. It creates a funnel, or holding area, slowing the movement of food into the main stomach. The goal is therefore not to aim to eat a particular amount of food to fill a small stomach, as this does not exist. Instead be guided by the feedback you are getting after each mouthful of food and stop as soon as you feel satisfied.

The amount of food appropriate for a meal following gastric band surgery remains controversial. As yet, the perfect serve size has not been established, hence people are told different things depending on the preference of their surgeon and support team. Some teams recommend a meal size of half a cup of food, some recommend one cup, others a bread and butter plate. (Note that one cup of diced food will generally fill the inside rim of a bread and butter plate when tipped out.)

The amount of food you require at each meal can vary and this will depend on the type of food you choose, how long ago you last ate, the time of the day, whether you are stressed or relaxed and many other factors.

Be guided by your surgical team on the serve size appropriate for you, but more importantly, how you feel when you eat. Most recipes in this book make approximately four, one cup serves, so can easily be adapted to make an appropriate serve size for you. If you share the meals with family or friends (who have not had weight loss surgery), they would generally require two serves of the recipe.

Fluid

For some time people with a gastric band have been advised to avoid eating and drinking at the same time. More recent research has shown this may not be necessary, however your personal experience is important.

People with a gastric band have different experiences when drinking with food. Some find that sipping fluid with a meal, particularly alcohol, allows them to eat a little more than normal. For those who chew very well, a little fluid with food may wash the food down, making it take longer to feel satisfied during a meal. Those who take large bites, or don't chew food well and try to 'wash' food down with fluid will likely end up with discomfort. This may cause a feeling that food is sitting in your throat and may cause regurgitation. Some people will try to clear blockages with fluid. This may help, or may backfire, resulting in regurgitation of the fluid, food or both.

If you are taking small bites, chewing well and eating slowly, some fluid during a meal should not be a problem. Experiment with the timing of food and fluid to see how it affects your comfort during eating, your satisfaction, hunger and the overall amount you eat. If drinking with food allows you to eat more, this is not the goal of surgery and you may need to look at your habits.

If you find it is better to avoid drinking whilst eating, make sure you sip regularly throughout the day to keep hydrated. Aim to include at least 1500mL (1½L) per day.

> "The band is shaped like a ring but functions like a funnel. Eat slowly, chew well."
> - Dr Helen Patroney, Bariatric GP -

Sleeve Gastrectomy Surgery

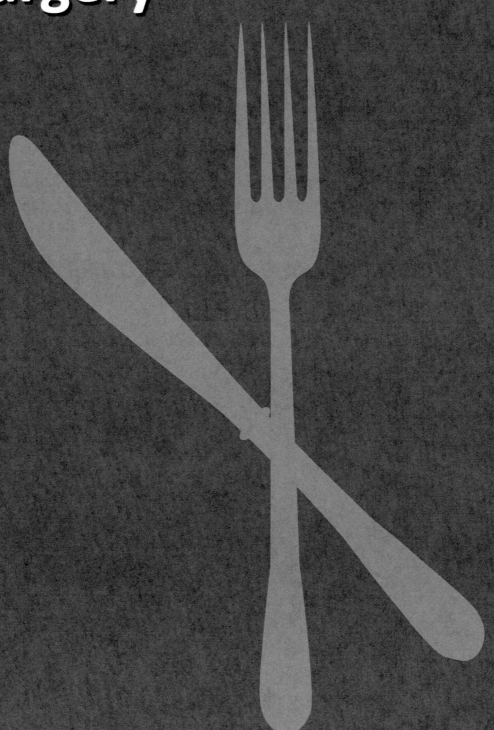

Sleeve Gastrectomy Surgery

How does sleeve gastrectomy surgery work?

Sleeve gastrectomy surgery reduces the size of the stomach by stapling along its length to form a long tube that looks similar to a banana. The majority of the stomach is then removed and discarded. The new banana shaped stomach is long and thin hence is often referred to as a 'sleeve'.

About 80-90% of the stomach is removed making it much smaller, hence it holds much less food than it did previously. This smaller stomach helps you feel satisfied after eating a small amount of food. In addition, the part of the stomach that is removed is the part that secretes much of the hormone called ghrelin, which is involved in stimulating appetite. It is thought that producing less ghrelin further helps to reduce hunger after surgery. Although ghrelin levels start to rise again after surgery, they don't seem to return to their previous levels and so hunger is more easily satisfied.

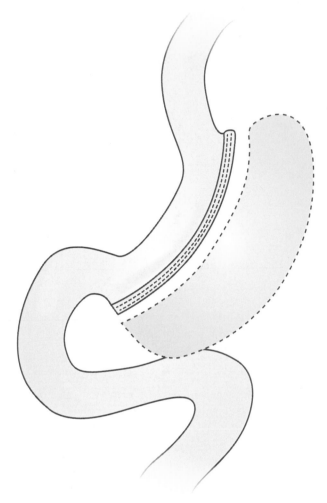

Sleeve Gastrectomy

Recovering from surgery

Following sleeve gastrectomy surgery there will be some swelling associated with creating the new, smaller stomach. You will therefore need to follow a recovery diet to allow your sleeve to heal. Details are discussed in the *Recovering From Surgery* section (page 52).

Maintenance

Whilst gastric band surgery requires ongoing adjustments, the sleeve does not require any adjustments. However, follow up is necessary to ensure your weight loss is on track, you are getting adequate nutrition and that the surgery is not having any negative effects on your health. Unlike

the adjustable gastric band the sleeve gastrectomy is not reversible. The stomach may stretch, or adapt to fit a little more food, but it cannot grow back. A sleeve gastrectomy therefore is a commitment for life.

As you will be eating less after sleeve gastrectomy, making the most of your food choices is important to help you obtain all the nutrients required for good health. Preventing nutrient deficiencies is discussed in detail in the *Nutritional Impacts of Weight Loss Surgery and Supplementation* chapter (page 232).

Following a sleeve gastrectomy most people will

lose most of their excess weight in the first year. After this time weight loss often stabilises, so make the most of this period by making good food choices and regular physical activity a habit for life. After the first year, your ongoing success will depend on your efforts to change your lifestyle and maintain these habits in the long term.

Whilst the size of the stomach changes after surgery, the type of foods that can be eaten does not. Choosing high-energy (calorie or kilojoule) foods regularly will hinder your progress. As with other types of weight loss surgery, snacking or grazing, lack of physical activity and poor food choices can lead to weight regain. Positive, lifelong changes to eating and physical activity will ensure your long-term success.

Poor food choices can also cause dumping syndrome. This is discussed in detail on page 223. Avoiding sugary foods will help prevent dumping syndrome.

Studies have found that those who had regular follow up after sleeve gastrectomy achieved better weight loss, health improvement, quality of life and food tolerance, than those who did not. Your support team is there to guide you to achieve the best results following surgery, so make the most of the team and keep in touch! They have all sorts of hints and tips to help you achieve success on your weight loss journey.

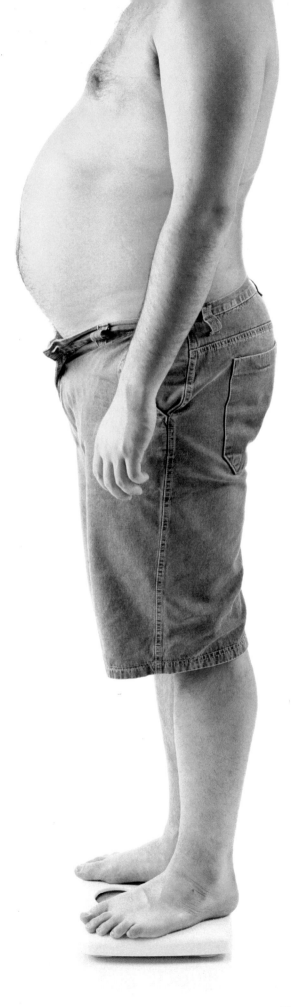

Eating and Drinking after Sleeve Gastrectomy Surgery

How much should I be eating?

An Australian study from Mercy Bariatrics in Perth, Western Australia, has investigated the average capacity, which is the amount of food that sleeves are able to hold. Immediately following surgery, a sleeve may only tolerate one quarter of a cup of food (or fluid food) at one time. Therefore, during the recovery stage, it is important to sip small amounts of fluid regularly. Over time your sleeve will get used to a little more food. At six months, you will manage about half a cup of food at a time. By 12 to 18 months you will manage about one cup of solid food. This is a guide only and will vary between people.

Sleeves come in different sizes or widths, depending on the preference of your surgeon. Over time and with experience, surgeons who perform sleeve gastrectomy surgeries have moved to smaller sleeve sizes. Sometimes a larger sleeve size will be chosen depending on your energy and fluid requirements. A smaller sleeve will generally hold less food than a larger sleeve and will not stretch as much over time. What is most important is to listen to the signals from your sleeve to find out how much food is right for you. Eat to a point where you feel satisfied; never eat past the point of feeling full. People with a sleeve often describe a feeling where they think they could probably fit in just one more mouthful. This is usually not the case and the extra mouthful causes discomfort. The aim is to eat until you are still comfortable. You will feel uncomfortable when you have eaten too much so try to stop eating before this feeling. To learn more about interpreting your satiety signals, see the hunger and satiety scale on page 104.

Our stomach is designed to stretch; hence a sleeve can also stretch. Regularly eating past the point of feeling satisfied could stretch the sleeve, which can hinder your success.

The amount you can tolerate will also vary according to the texture of food you eat. It is likely that you will tolerate more food if it is in a liquid form, rather than a solid form. For example, you will generally tolerate more of a chicken and vegetable soup than grilled chicken and steamed vegetables.

Solid food will tend to sit in the stomach longer than liquid, so once you have recovered, try to limit liquid meals. Choose solid foods most of the time to help you feel satisfied for a longer time after eating.

Fluid

Keeping hydrated in the early stages following sleeve gastrectomy can be challenging. Sometimes the swelling associated with having surgery makes it difficult to drink and keep fluids down. Try the following to increase your fluid intake:

- Water can be difficult for some people immediately after surgery as it feels "heavy". Try adding a small dash of juice, diet cordial or slice of lemon.

- Start slowly and drink small amounts. Try 40-50ml spaced out over 30 minutes and increase the amount as you feel able.

- Sit upright when drinking. If you are able, walk around between drinks.

- Try drinks at different temperatures. You may find cold or hot fluids more comfortable than those at room temperature. Herbal teas are generally tolerated well.

- Choose very thin fluids in the initial stages as these are often easier to manage. Dilute thicker fluids such as smoothies and soups with milk, water or ice.

- Freeze nourishing liquids such as smoothies,

milk drinks or VLED milkshakes into ice blocks and suck on them slowly over time.

- Some people may find rehydration solutions, such as Hydralyte®, may be beneficial to increase hydration.

Avoid drinking high-energy fluids such as commercial milkshakes, flavoured coffees, regular flavoured milks and large quantities of juices. These will add too many calories or kilojoules and provide very little satiety, which is the feeling of satisfaction after eating. They can therefore interfere with your weight loss.

Carbonated or 'fizzy' drinks are generally not well tolerated soon after surgery, causing pain and discomfort and putting too much pressure on your new stomach. Therefore it is best to avoid them.

If you are not getting enough fluid (or as much as you did prior to surgery) you may feel lightheaded or dizzy. When this happens you should sit or lay down until you feel more comfortable.

Following surgery your new, smaller stomach or sleeve cannot fit both food and fluid at one time so try to separate food and fluid by about 30 minutes. It is also difficult to guzzle large amounts of fluid at one time, so you will need to drink small amounts regularly. Make it a habit to sip fluids throughout the day. Remind yourself to drink often; carry a water bottle with you, keep a jug of water on your desk at work or in a place where you walk past it often at home. If you find plain water difficult try herbal tea or add diet cordial to water. Try to drink at least 1500mL (1½L) of fluid daily.

Cranberry, Raspberry and Strawberry iced tea. Brew with hot water, chill and serve in a tall glass with ice, lime wedges and/or mint leaves (as pictured).

Gastric Bypass Surgery

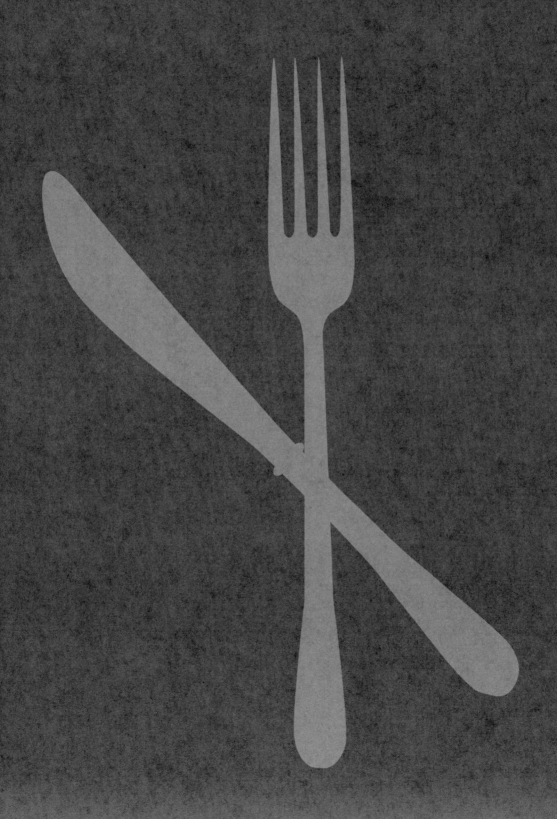

Gastric Bypass Surgery
Roux-en-Y Gastric Bypass

How does gastric bypass surgery work?

During Roux-en-Y gastric bypass surgery (gastric bypass) the top of the stomach is stapled to form a small pouch. The small pouch becomes a new, smaller stomach and is totally separate to the rest of the stomach. This small pouch is then 're-plumbed' to the jejunum, the middle part of the small intestine, bypassing the first part of the intestine called the duodenum.

The new, smaller stomach pouch allows you to eat only a small amount of food before feeling satisfied. There are also some hormonal changes that occur similar to those described following sleeve gastrectomy. Gastric bypass surgery, however, causes further hormonal changes that are also known to decrease your appetite.

It is important to note that bypassing the first part of the intestine means less vitamins and minerals are absorbed. This is discussed in detail in the *Nutritional Impacts of Weight Loss Surgery and Supplementation* chapter (page 232).

Recovering from surgery

Following gastric bypass surgery there will be some swelling associated with creating the new, smaller stomach and the 're-plumbing' to the small intestine. You will therefore need to follow a recovery diet to allow healing to occur. Details are discussed in the *Recovering From Surgery* section (page 52).

Maintenance

Unlike the gastric band, the gastric bypass does not require any ongoing adjustments. However, follow up is necessary to ensure your weight loss is appropriate, you are receiving adequate nutrition

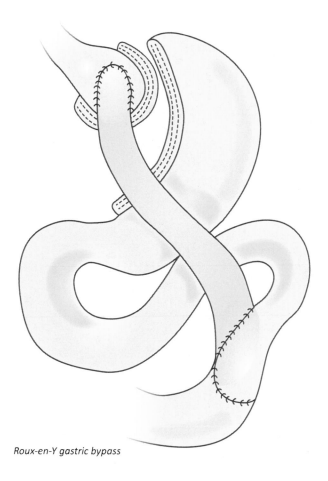

Roux-en-Y gastric bypass

and that the surgery is not having any negative effects on your health.

One study has found the most intense weight loss occurs in the first six months following gastric bypass surgery and will slow in the second six months, stabilising in the second year. It is likely, however, that everyone will have a different experience.

As with all forms of weight loss surgery, success is not guaranteed. Lifestyle changes including healthy eating and regular physical activity are key ingredients in your long term success following surgery. Whilst the size of the new stomach helps prevent overeating, the food choices you make are important. People who maintain their weight losses long term generally avoid high fat, high-energy foods.

As well as improving weight loss and maintenance, it is important to avoid high sugar and/or high fat foods as following gastric bypass surgery they can lead to a side effect called dumping syndrome. Dumping syndrome is discussed in the *Troubleshooting and Common Complaints* chapter (page 216).

Studies have shown that following gastric bypass surgery, those who kept in closest contact with their support team achieved better results. Your team is there to guide you to get the best results following surgery, so make the most of them and keep in touch! They have all sorts of hints and tips to help you on a successful journey.

One Anastomosis Gastric Bypass

During the one anastomosis gastric bypass (also referred to the omega loop or "mini-gastric bypass"), the size of the normal stomach is reduced by separating a tube-like pouch of stomach from the rest of the stomach. This tubular pouch is then connected (anastomosed) to the intestine, bypassing up to 200cm of the upper part of the intestine. This is different from the traditional Roux-en-Y bypass which requires two connections (anastomoses).

The new, smaller stomach pouch allows you to eat a smaller amount of food before feeling satisfied. As part of the intestine is bypassed, less food is absorbed, further assisting you to lose weight. It is important to note that bypassing part of the intestine means not only less food is absorbed, but also less vitamins and minerals.

Similarly to the Roux-en-Y bypass, there will be some swelling associated with creating the new, smaller stomach and the 're-plumbing' to the intestine. You will therefore need to follow a recovery diet to allow healing to occur. Details are discussed in the *Recovering From Surgery* section (page 52).

Long term follow up is again necessary to ensure your weight loss is appropriate, you are receiving adequate nutrition and that the surgery is not having any negative effects on your health.

As the nutritional management of both the Roux-en-Y and one anastomosis surgeries is similar, from here on, this book will simply refer to gastric bypass surgery.

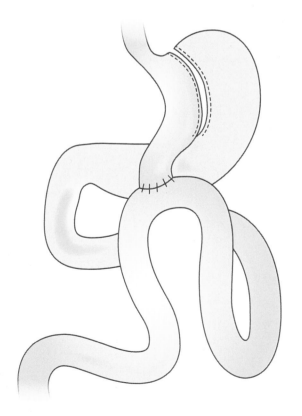

One Anastomosis Gastric Bypass

Eating and Drinking after Gastric Bypass

How much should I be eating?

The optimal meal size, or amount of food that can be eaten at one time, has not been well researched after gastric bypass surgery. Surgeons will have a different way of performing the surgery, hence will create stomach pouches of different sizes. Whilst some may only tolerate one quarter of a cup in the initial stage, in general, most people will tolerate half a cup of food or fluid in the early stages after surgery. This may increase to approximately one cup between six to twelve months after surgery. This is a guide only and will vary between people.

There will also be variation in how much a new stomach pouch will stretch after surgery. Because the stomach is designed to stretch, it is common for the new stomach pouch to stretch after a few years. As the stomach stretches, the feeling of satiety (or satisfaction) after eating a small amount of food can decrease.

When you eat past the point of feeling satisfied and start to feel 'full', you will reach a point where one more bite will cause discomfort and possibly nausea. This is a sign you have eaten too much. Try to stop eating once you feel satisfied, or no longer hungry.

As no single serving size can be recommended for all people following gastric bypass, it is up to you to judge the amount of food that makes you satisfied. Most recipes in this book make approximately four, one cup serves, so can easily be adapted to make an appropriate serve size for you. If you share the meals with family or friends (without a gastric bypass), they would generally require two serves of the recipe.

The amount you can tolerate will also vary according to the texture of food you eat. It is likely that you will tolerate more food if it is in a liquid form, rather than a solid form. For example, you will generally tolerate more of a chicken and vegetable soup than grilled chicken and steamed vegetables.

Solid food will tend to sit in the stomach longer than liquid, so once you have recovered, try to limit liquid meals. Choose solid foods most of the time to help you feel satisfied for longer after eating.

Fluid

Following surgery your new, smaller stomach cannot fit both food and fluid at one time, so try to separate food and fluid by about 30 minutes. It is also difficult to guzzle large amounts of fluid at one time, so you will need to drink small amounts regularly. Make it a habit to sip fluids throughout the day. Remind yourself to drink often; carry a water bottle with you, keep a jug of water on your desk at work or in a place where you walk past it often at home. If you find plain water difficult try herbal tea or add diet cordial to water. Try to drink at least 1500mL (1½L) of fluid daily.

> "Having a small stomach pouch is a tool that can serve you well your entire life, but you must learn to use it properly."
>
> - Colleen, gastric bypass -

Preparing for Surgery

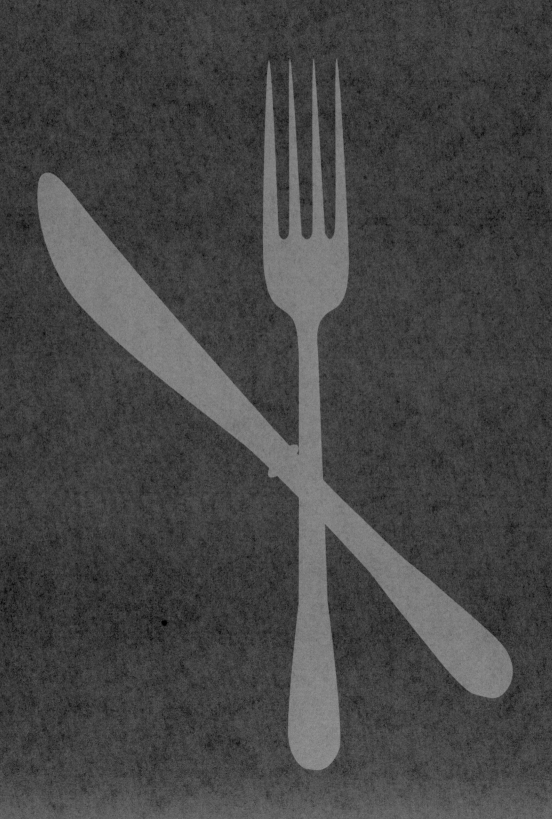

Preparing the Body for Surgery

Very low energy diet programs

Once you have made the commitment to have weight loss surgery, preparing your body for surgery is important to make sure the surgery is less complicated for the surgeon and safer for you.

People store fat all over the body, including inside the liver and around the stomach. When the surgeon comes to operate, the liver must be moved aside so the stomach can be accessed. A liver that is storing too much fat becomes very large and can be difficult to move during surgery, similar to moving a lump of jelly with chopsticks. Further, a large amount of fat around the stomach makes it hard to see and makes access to the stomach more difficult. Hence it is useful to reduce the size of the liver and the fat around the stomach before surgery and a very low energy diet is recommended as the best way to do this.

A Very Low Energy Diet (VLED) or Very Low Calorie Diet (VLCD) is low in energy (calories or kilojoules). When you gain little energy from food, the body has to find energy from elsewhere to perform all of its normal functions. This energy is found in stored body fat, some of which is stored in the organs, including the liver. Therefore a VLED program promotes weight loss and helps organs such as the liver reduce in size.

A smaller liver is easier for the surgeon to move and is less likely to be damaged. Other benefits of losing weight prior to surgery include reduced operating time, improved recovery, improved mobility following surgery and potentially improved management of other medical conditions such as diabetes or high blood pressure.

One of the most commonly used programs is the Optifast VLCD®. The Optifast VLCD® was used in the original research that showed a VLED can reduce liver volume and cause it to shrink. However, there are other high quality products such as KicStart® VLCD and Dr. MacLeod's® which would likely have a similar effect. Always check with your team before choosing an alternative product.

If your surgeon does not recommend you follow a VLED program, discuss this with them, as these programs are safe and beneficial for most people. A dietitian and GP should supervise the program, particularly if you have a medical condition such as type 2 diabetes or high blood pressure.

If you don't have a dietitian, ask your surgeon to refer you to one. Alternatively, find one locally that is both an Accredited Practising Dietitian and specialises in weight loss surgery using the Obesity Surgery Society of Australia and New Zealand (OSSANZ) website: www.ossanz.com.au. Just as you wouldn't undergo a knee or hip replacement without the support of a physiotherapist, weight loss surgery involves input from the wider allied health team. Recruit support from your wider health team; speak with your bariatric dietitian, exercise physiologist, psychologist, diabetes educator and GP to support you in the journey.

What are VLED programs?

The VLED products are meal replacement products that provide the body with essential vitamins, minerals and protein. The products are generally available in four forms, depending on the brand:

- milkshakes
- soups
- bars
- desserts.

The various forms of VLED products are virtually the same nutritionally, hence you can vary them to suit your taste.

As a minimum you should replace three meals per day with a VLED product. Obtaining adequate protein is essential whilst following a VLED to avoid muscle breakdown. To achieve this, many people will need more than three VLED products daily. This can be discussed with your dietitian.

During a VLED program you should also eat 'low energy foods' which are listed on page 28. Low energy foods provide fibre, vitamins and minerals, but very little energy (calories or kilojoules) whilst on the program. These foods are the basis for the recipes used in the *Low Energy Vegetables* recipes (from page 33). Low energy foods can also be used as snacks, or if you wish to create your own recipes.

There is a range of benefits in including vegetables and salads in addition to the VLED products. Including vegetables or salads helps you feel more satisfied on the VLED program and increases fibre, vitamin and mineral intake. To further increase your fibre intake you can include a fibre supplement such as Benefiber®. It is also appropriate to include a multivitamin and mineral supplement on a VLED program, particularly if you are following the program for more than two weeks.

"Be adventurous to stave off boredom with the food. I roasted capsicums and eggplant and added my olive oil allowance, garlic and vinegar and pretended I was in Rome."
- *Robby, gastric band* -

LOW ENERGY FOODS

Low Energy Vegetables

- alfalfa sprouts
- asparagus
- bok choy
- broccoli
- brussels sprouts
- celery
- cabbage
- capsicum
- carrots
- cauliflower
- cucumber
- eggplant
- green beans
- lettuce
- leeks
- mushrooms
- onion
- radishes
- shallots
- silver beet
- snow peas
- spinach
- squash
- tomato
- watercress
- zucchini

Herbs and Spices

- allspice
- basil
- cardamom
- celery flakes
- chilli
- chives
- cinnamon
- cloves
- coriander
- cumin
- curry powder
- dill
- fennel
- garlic
- ginger
- mint
- mustard seed
- nutmeg
- oregano
- paprika
- parsley
- pepper
- rosemary
- sage
- thyme
- turmeric
- tarragon

Soups

- reduced salt stock cubes or powder
- Bonox® (in moderation)
- miso soup
- vegetable soups (made using stock powder, low energy vegetables and herbs/spices only)

Sauces and Condiments

- lemon juice
- lime juice
- vinegar - all varieties
- Worcestershire sauce
- reduced salt soy sauce
- mustard
- tomato paste
- diet, oil free or fat free salad dressings

LOW ENERGY FOODS

Miscellaneous

- oil - 1 teaspoon per day
- artificial sweeteners
- unsweetened lollies or gum
- diet jelly
- essence: almond, aniseed, brandy, coconut, lemon, orange, peppermint, rum

Low Energy Fluids

- water
- diet cordial
- soda water
- plain mineral water
- tea & coffee* (no or 30ml skim milk and no sugar)
- herbal teas
- diet soft drink

A small amount of caffeine can be included in the form of 1-2 cups of coffee per day.

Side effects of a VLED program

A VLED causes the body to burn your fat stores for 'fuel'. When we burn our fat stores we produce chemicals called ketones in a process called ketosis. Ketosis helps reduce appetite and prevents the loss of lean muscle tissue as you lose weight, which is helpful on a VLED. However, you are likely to experience a 'three day challenge' when you first begin the program. As the body systems move into ketosis, some people experience fatigue, hunger, headaches, nausea and lack of concentration. Keep focused and positive during the three-day challenge, knowing it will soon pass and these side effects will subside.

When a VLED is used for two weeks prior to surgery, significant side effects are unlikely. If you continue a VLED for longer than this, side effects that may occur include:

- sensitivity to cold
- dry skin
- temporary rash
- temporary hair loss
- low blood pressure on standing
- fatigue
- diarrhoea
- constipation
- muscle cramps
- bad breath
- irritability
- menstrual disturbances.

Constipation is one side effect that can be managed. If constipation becomes a problem, ensure you are including plenty of low energy vegetables and plenty of water. Check the nutrition information panel to see if the VLED products you are using have fibre added. If not, you could look for an alternative product that does. Alternatively, you could try Benefiber® which is colourless and tasteless and can be added to VLED shakes or soups without altering the flavour.

An adequate fluid intake also helps prevent constipation. You should include an additional two litres of low energy fluid per day above that in the VLED milkshakes or soups. Avoid alcohol on the VLED program as it is high in energy (calories or kilojoules). Limit caffeine; a small amount of caffeine can be included in the form of one to two cups of coffee per day.

If you are used to drinking large amounts of regular soft drink, milk drinks or coffee and are finding it hard to drink an additional two litres of fluid, try some of the following ideas:

- Splash diet cordial concentrate, such as diet blackcurrant or diet lime into soda water.
- Add a dash of lemon juice or wedge of fresh lemon to diet tonic.
- Add a wedge of fresh lime or lime juice to diet ginger ale.
- Make your own iced tea by brewing herbal tea with hot water, then chilling. Serve in a tall glass with ice, sliced lemon and fresh mint.
- Try fruity herbal teas such as cranberry, raspberry and strawberry. If you are a liquorice lover, try the aniseed varieties.
- Add a squirt of pure lemon or lime juice to water or soda water for a refreshing change.
- Add more vegetables to your day with the Lemon & Greens Smoothie (page 49) or Spicy Vegetable Smoothie (page 47).

When a VLED program is used for two weeks prior to surgery you will not need extensive follow up. If you continue a VLED program for longer than this, regular monitoring by your GP or bariatric dietitian is essential. If you are on medications your GP may need to review them, as you may need to decrease doses whilst using a VLED. This is particularly important if you are on medication for, or use insulin to manage diabetes.

Purchasing VLED products

Most pharmacies stock Optifast VLCD® or can order it for you. Shop around for competitive prices such as the 'warehouse' or 'discount' pharmacies, or if you have membership cards with a particular pharmacy chain you may be able to receive a discount. Some may find it cheaper or more convenient to order Optifast VLCD® from online pharmacies.

To purchase KicStart® VLCD go to: www.healthyweightforlife.com.au.

To purchase Dr. MacLeod's® go to: www.DrMacLeods.com.au.

Hints and tips for using VLED products

- Use very cold water and ice cubes to mix milkshakes.
- If the texture of milkshakes is too thick when mixed according to the packet directions, add extra water.
- Mix milkshakes in a plastic shaker or use a blender/milkshake maker to ensure they mix well.
- Flavour milkshakes by adding a teaspoon of coffee (preferably decaf), diet ice cream topping, diet jelly crystals, or flavour essences such as almond, aniseed, brandy, coconut, lemon, orange, peppermint or rum. For example:
  - add coffee to chocolate milkshakes for a mocha flavour
  - add coconut essence to chocolate milkshakes for a coconut rough
  - add almond or hazelnut essence to chocolate or vanilla milkshakes for a nutty change
  - add lemon or orange essence to vanilla milkshakes for a fruity twist.
- Freeze milkshakes in summer and eat with a spoon.
- Dissolve milkshake powder in a small amount of water, and then blend with ice cubes to make a 'slushie'.
- Freeze Optifast VLCD® dessert for 30 minutes for an ice cream consistency.
- Serve Optifast VLCD® chocolate dessert with diet chocolate or strawberry topping. Alternatively, add a drop of peppermint essence during preparation and garnish with mint leaves to serve.
- Add chopped vegetables to soups, for example:
  - frozen mixed vegetables
  - cooked, blended cauliflower
  - asparagus cuts and tips (drained)
  - roasted red capsicum, skin removed.
- Add a flavour hit to soups with fresh or dried herbs and/or curry powder.

"I am a huge fan of the Optifast VLCD® Lemon Crème and Chocolate Mousse Desserts. I put them in the freezer to make them harder like ice cream."

- Lisi, gastric bypass -

VLED SAMPLE MENU

Breakfast

1 VLED bar or milkshake

Lunch

1 VLED bar, milkshake or soup

PLUS low energy vegetables or salad, for example:

- Mixed Vegetable Soup (page 35)
- Vietnamese Coleslaw (page 37)
- Spanish Salad (page 39)
- Tossed Vegetable Salad (page 41)
- Asian Carrot Salad (page 43)
- Mushroom Salad (page 44).

Dinner

1 VLED bar, milkshake or soup

PLUS low energy vegetables or salad, for example:

- Baby Spinach with Lemon (page 40)
- Mixed Vegetable Stir-fry (page 34)
- Broccoli with Fennel (page 50)
- Vegetable Kebabs (page 45)
- Ratatouille (page 42)
- Roasted Balsamic Asparagus & Mushrooms (page 48)
- Cauliflower & Cabbage Curry (page 46)
- Vegetable Stack (page 38).

Snacks

If you are hungry between meals, try some of the following options:

- Raw vegetable sticks with fat free tomato salsa
- Diet jelly
- Mixed Vegetable Soup (page 35)
- Spicy Vegetable Smoothie (page 47)
- Lemon & Greens Smoothie (page 49)
- Cauliflower Popcorn (page 51)
- Kale Chips (page 51).

Please note: As explained on page 26 - 27, many people will need more than three VLED products per day to get adequate protein and this should be discussed with your dietitian. These additional products could therefore also be included between meals. Also try to include two litres of low energy fluid in addition to the VLED products themselves.

Using the Low Energy Vegetable Recipes

The Low Energy Vegetables can be included at meal times, in addition to a serve of your chosen VLED product.

If you would like to experiment with various salads and vegetables to create your own low energy vegetable recipes, refer to the list of 'allowed' low energy foods provided on page 28. You could also use these ingredients to create vegetable smoothies. For inspiration see the Lemon & Greens Smoothie (page 49) and the Spicy Vegetable Smoothie (page 47).

Some of the recipes are suitable to freeze and this is indicated where appropriate.

Serve sizes

Each low energy vegetable recipe indicates how many serves it makes, either two or four. This allows you to share the dishes with family or friends. They may include the vegetable recipes as a side dish with a protein-containing food such as meat, chicken, fish, eggs, legumes or tofu. Note that as these recipes are for use prior to surgery, the serve sizes are larger than they would be following surgery.

Hints and tips

Throughout the recipes, practical hints and tips are included between the yellow lines.

"We were both eating these recipes. My husband was never a vege person but he liked these."
- Marie, gastric band -

"Having been on VLED previously (and struggled), I found it much easier and more enjoyable this time around. The difference was combining the VLED with your great recipes. Thank you, without the recipes I very much doubt I could have lasted 3 weeks on a VLED alone!"
- Alison, gastric bypass -

"I tried a lot of the salads on the VLED stage, they were really nice."
- Julie, gastric band -

"I had my gastric sleeve in January 2011 and I don't know where I'd be without your book. Pre op - the ratatouille saved me!!!!!"
- Kate, sleeve gastrectomy -

"I was amazed how good these recipes were! At no stage on the pre-op diet did I feel hungry."
- Geoff, gastric band -

"My first day on the pre-op diet I tried the Ratatouille from Sally's book. Yum! I'm not going to starve that's for sure!"
- Courtney, gastric bypass -

Mixed Vegetable Stir-fry

Serves 4

Oil spray

1 onion, sliced

1 clove garlic, crushed

1 red chilli, finely diced

1 teaspoon ginger, finely grated

1 green capsicum, sliced

2 red capsicums, sliced

2 cups mushrooms, sliced

1 stalk celery, chopped

2 cups snow peas or green beans, sliced

1 tablespoon soy sauce

Freshly ground black pepper to taste

Heat a non-stick frying pan or wok that has been sprayed with oil. Add onion and cook for a few minutes. Add garlic, ginger and chilli and cook until fragrant. Add remaining vegetables and stir-fry over medium heat until vegetables are cooked to the desired tenderness. Whilst vegetables are cooking, stir through the soy sauce. Season with pepper to taste.

Nutrition information (per serve): kilojoules 310, calories 74, protein 5g, fat 1.5g, saturated fat negligible, carbohydrate 7.5g, fibre 4g.

- Including a range of different coloured vegetables is important. Different colours indicate that they contain different nutrients.
- For family and friends, stir-fry some lean beef or chicken strips and serve with some rice or noodles.
- Try serving with konjac rice or konjac noodles. Do not use regular pasta or noodles on the very low energy diet.

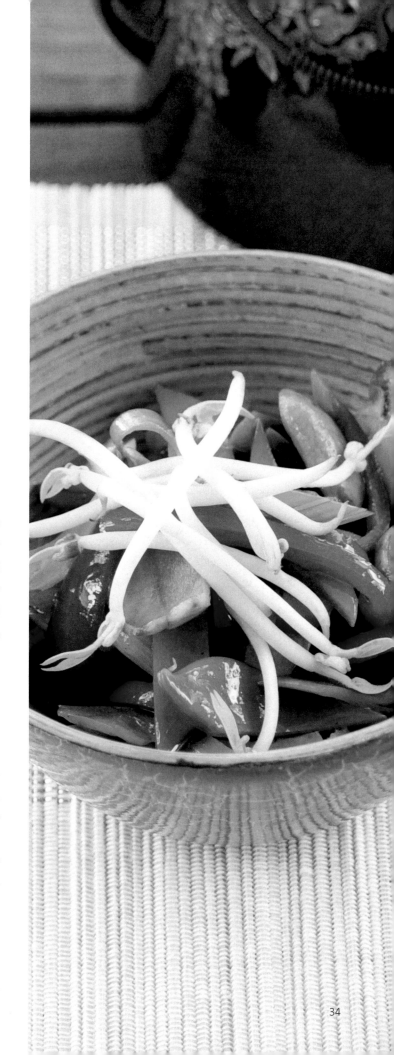

Mixed Vegetable Soup

Serves 4

Oil spray

2 cloves garlic, crushed

5 cups salt reduced chicken or vegetable stock

1 carrot, peeled and diced

1 onion, diced

½ zucchini, diced

¼ cabbage, chopped

1 cup green beans, chopped

¼ cauliflower, finely diced

2 tablespoons no added salt tomato paste

400g no added salt, chopped tinned tomatoes

1 teaspoon dried basil

1 teaspoon dried oregano

Freshly ground black pepper to taste

Heat a saucepan that has been sprayed with oil. Add the carrots, onion and garlic and cook for about 5 minutes. Add all the remaining ingredients except the zucchini and bring to the boil. Cover, reduce the heat to medium and simmer for about 15 minutes or until the beans are tender. Add the zucchini and cook until zucchini is tender. If you like a chunky soup, serve as is. Otherwise, blend in a food processor or blender until smooth. Season with pepper to taste.

Nutrition information (per serve): kilojoules 405, calories 97, protein 4.5g, fat 2.5g, saturated fat 0.5g, carbohydrate 11g, fibre 6.5g.

Suitable to freeze.

> "This has been really handy. I kept some in the freezer, it's very filling."
> *- Janneke, gastric band -*

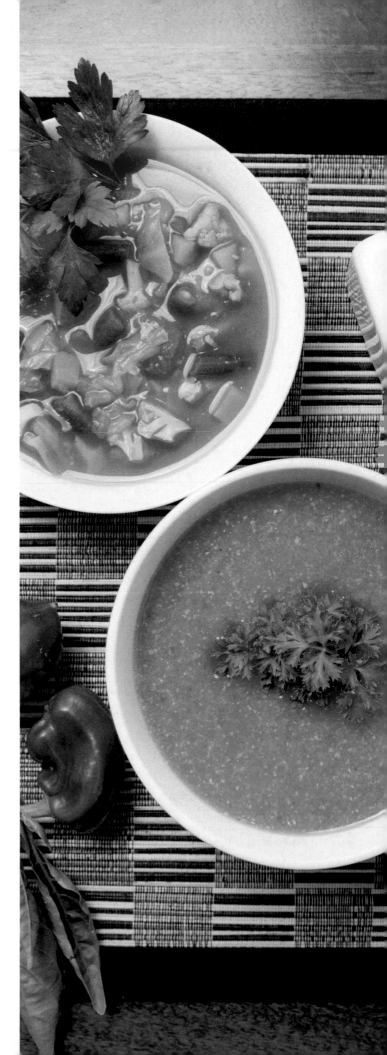

Oven Roasted Vegetable Salad

Serves 4

Oil spray

2 eggplant, diced

2 zucchini, diced

2 red capsicums, diced

2 cloves garlic, crushed

2 cups mushrooms, diced

2 cups cherry tomatoes, halved

2 cups baby spinach

Seasoning

¼ cup fresh flat-leaf parsley, chopped

¼ cup fresh basil, chopped

2 teaspoons lemon rind, finely grated

2 cloves garlic, crushed

1-2 tablespoons balsamic vinegar (optional)

Preheat oven to 200°C. Combine eggplant, zucchini, capsicum and garlic in a small, shallow baking dish. Spray with oil. Roast uncovered for 30 minutes, stirring occasionally. Add mushroom and tomatoes and roast uncovered for about 10 minutes or until vegetables are just tender.Meanwhile, combine ingredients for seasoning.Combine seasoning, vegetables and baby spinach in a bowl. Stir well to coat.

Nutrition information (per serve): kilojoules 370, calories 89, protein 5g, fat 2g, saturated fat negligible, carbohydrate 8.5g, fibre 7.5g.

Serve as a hot salad or refrigerate and take to work as a cold salad for lunch.

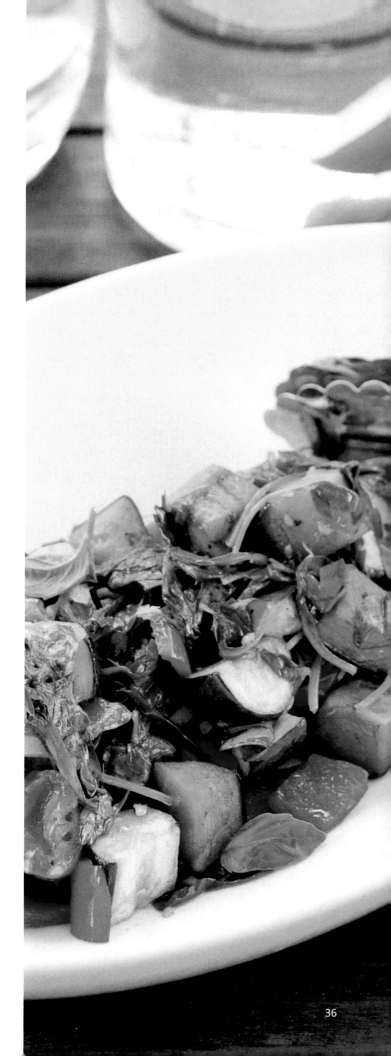

Vietnamese Coleslaw

Serves 4

2 carrots

1 cup green cabbage, shredded

1½ cups red cabbage, shredded

1 yellow capsicum, sliced thinly

1 cup bean sprouts

2 spring onions, thinly sliced

¼ cup loosely packed fresh coriander leaves

Dressing

¼ cup lime juice

1 clove garlic, crushed

1 tablespoon salt reduced soy sauce (optional)

Using a vegetable peeler, slice carrot into ribbons. Place in a medium bowl with cabbages, capsicum, sprouts, onion and coriander and toss gently to combine. Combine ingredients for dressing in a screw-top jar and shake well. Drizzle over salad.

Nutrition information (per serve): kilojoules 195, calories 47, protein 3g, fat 0.5g, saturated fat negligible, carbohydrate 5g, fibre 4.5g.

This recipe makes a great side dish when you progress to the *Recipes for Healthy Living*. It provides a fresh alternative to the creamy varieties of coleslaw that are generally high in fat.

> "I really enjoyed this one."
>
> *- Wayne, gastric band -*

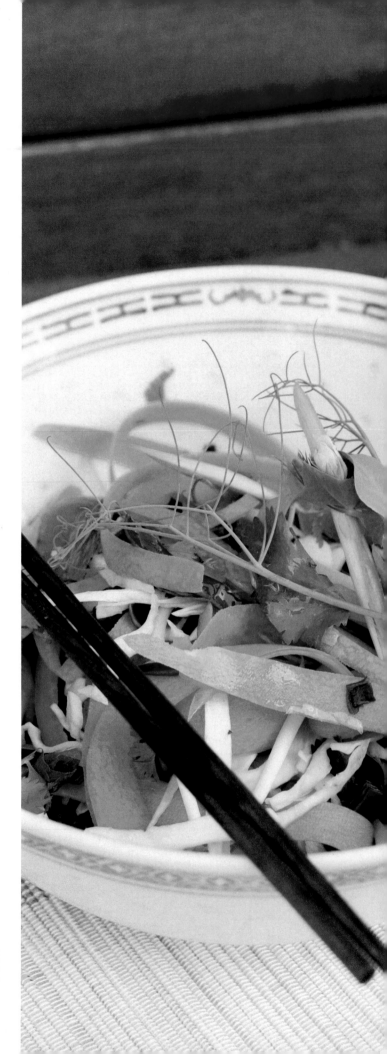

Vegetable Stack

Serves 4

2 red capsicums, sliced into flat pieces

1 eggplant, thinly sliced

2 zucchini, thinly sliced

1 onions, thinly sliced

3 tomatoes, thinly sliced

3 cups mushrooms, thinly sliced

½ cup no added salt, crushed tinned tomatoes

Preheat oven to 180°C. Lay 4 pieces of foil flat, approximately 20cm x 20cm or use an oven proof lasagne tray to make 1 larger stack. Layer vegetables in any desired order to form a stack in the centre of the foil. Pour crushed tomatoes over the top of the stack. Fold foil to enclose the stack forming a parcel. Bake in oven for approximately 30 minutes or until vegetables reach the desired tenderness. If baking as one large stack in a lasagne tray, you may need to double the cooking time.

Nutrition information (per serve): kilojoules 355, calories 85, protein 6g, fat 1g, saturated fat negligible, carbohydrate 10g, fibre 6.5g.

- At any stage of stacking, sprinkle with black pepper, basil or oregano for added flavour.
- The individual foil parcels can also be cooked on the barbeque, which is useful if hosting or attending a barbeque whilst on the VLED program.
- Following surgery add some protein with some wedges of firm, reduced fat ricotta or haloumi for a tasty vegetarian dish.

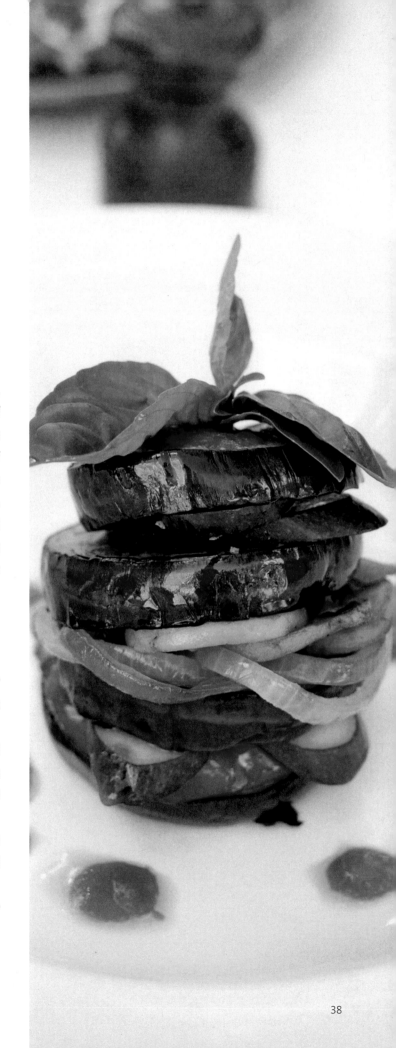

Spanish Salad

Serves 4

2 cucumbers, peeled and diced

4 tomatoes, seeded and diced

1 onion, finely chopped

2 green capsicums, chopped

Freshly ground black pepper

Dressing

2 cloves garlic, mashed

½ teaspoon ground cumin

2 tablespoons white vinegar

2 tablespoons parsley, chopped

2 spring onions, chopped

2 tablespoons lemon juice

Combine cucumber, tomato, onion and green capsicum in a bowl. Sprinkle with pepper. Combine dressing ingredients in a jar and shake to mix well. Pour over salad.

Nutrition information (per serve): kilojoules 270, calories 65, protein 3.5g, fat 0.5g, saturated fat negligible, carbohydrate 8.5g, fibre 4g.

"That was nice."

- Malcolm, gastric band -

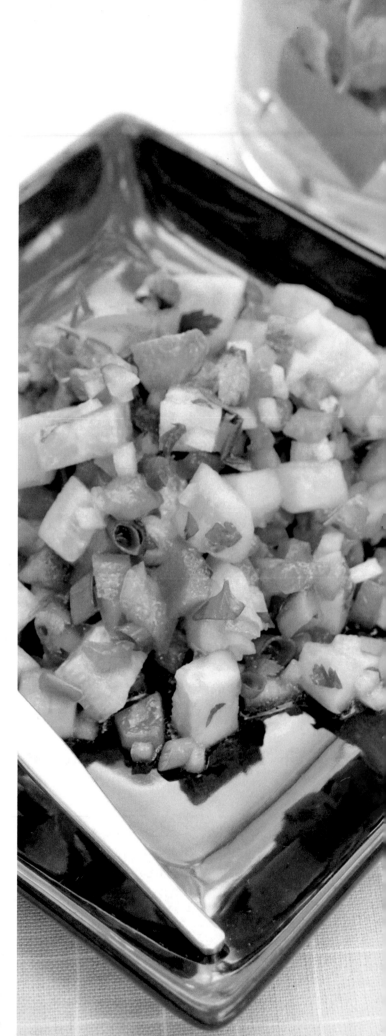

Baby Spinach with Lemon

Serves 2

½ cup salt reduced chicken stock

1 onion, sliced or diced

1 yellow capsicum, sliced or diced

1 clove garlic, crushed

2 teaspoons lemon zest

1 packet fresh baby spinach

Freshly ground black pepper

Heat a splash of chicken stock in a large frying pan on medium to high heat. When it starts to simmer, add the onion and capsicum. Cook until just beginning to soften, adding splashes of chicken stock to prevent burning. Add the garlic and lemon zest and stir for a minute or so. Add the spinach in handfuls, stirring into the hot mixture, adding more stock as needed. When all the spinach is added, cook until still bright green but fully cooked. Season with pepper to taste.

Nutrition information (per serve): kilojoules 245, calories 59, protein 4.5g, fat 0.5g, saturated fat negligible, carbohydrate 6g, fibre 4.5g.

"Really really nice."

- Amanda, gastric band -

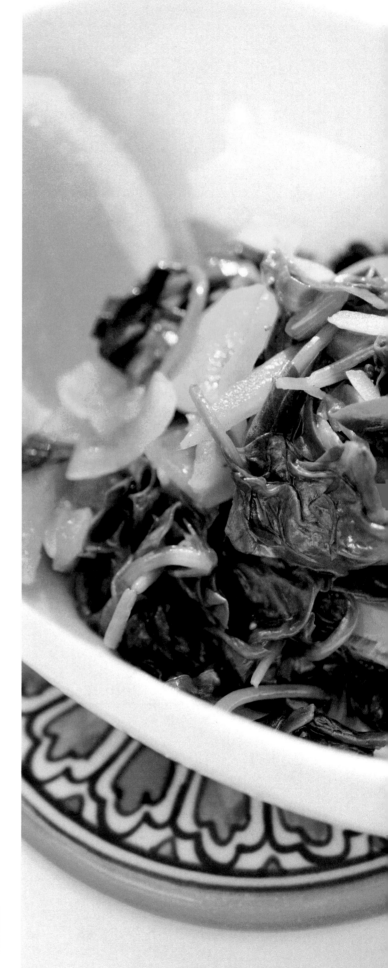

Tossed Vegetable Salad

Serves 4

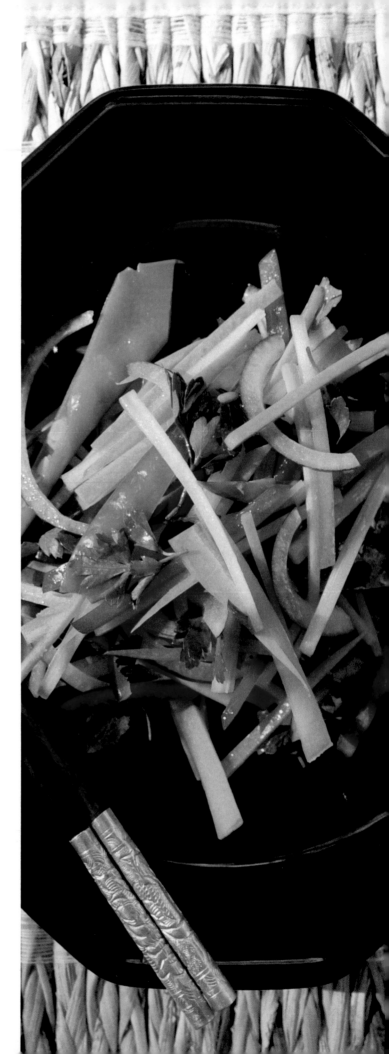

2 cups snow peas

2 carrots, thinly sliced

2 sticks celery, thinly sliced

1 red capsicum, cut into strips

½ red onion, cut into slices and separated into rings

¼ cup parsley, finely chopped

2 tablespoons fat free French dressing

½ cup radishes, thinly sliced

Combine snow peas, carrot, celery, capsicum, onion and parsley in a bowl. Toss with enough French dressing to moisten. Add radishes just before serving.

A simple recipe that can be used as a side dish in the future when you progress to the *Recipes for Healthy Living*. This is also a great base for a quick and easy lunch following surgery. Just combine with some tinned tuna or salmon in spring water, or some cooked kidney beans, butter beans or chickpeas.

Nutrition information (per serve): kilojoules 195, calories 47, protein 2g, fat negligible, saturated fat negligible, carbohydrate 7.5g, fibre 3g.

Ratatouille

Serves 4

Oil spray

1 onion, chopped

1 clove garlic, crushed

1 red capsicum, diced

1 stick celery, diced

2 cups mushrooms, diced

2 zucchini, diced

1 eggplant, diced

¼ cup fresh basil, chopped

400g no added salt, chopped tinned tomatoes

Heat a frying pan that has been sprayed with oil. Add onion, garlic, capsicum, celery and mushrooms. Sauté until vegetables are tender. Remove and set aside. Spray frying pan with oil again, add the zucchini and eggplant and saute until softened. Return capsicum mixture to frying pan. Add basil and tomatoes and simmer 5 minutes over low heat, stirring occasionally.

Nutrition information (per serve): kilojoules 335, calories 80, protein 4.5g, fat 2g, saturated fat negligible, carbohydrate 9g, fibre 5.5g.

- This recipe can be used as a sauce for other vegetables, or served as a sauce with meat, chicken or fish if eating with family or friends.
- This recipe is suitable to freeze.
- This dish makes a great 'pasta' sauce - use zucchini ribbons or konjac noodles as 'pasta'. Do not use regular pasta or noodles on the very low energy diet.

> **"I made this the most, we loved it."**
>
> *- Marie, gastric band -*

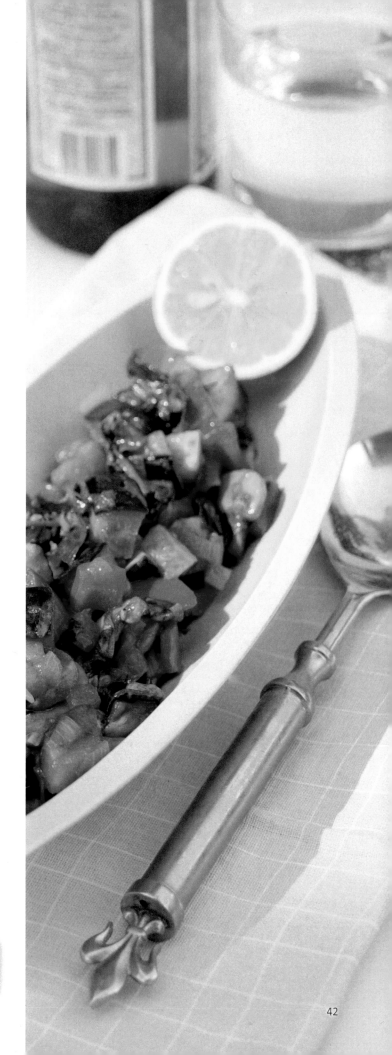

Asian Carrot Salad

Serves 4

2 carrots, peeled

1½ cups snow peas, thinly sliced diagonally

2 Lebanese cucumbers

1½ cups bean sprouts, trimmed

Dressing

2 tablespoons rice wine or white wine vinegar

2 teaspoons sesame oil

1 tablespoon salt reduced soy sauce

Freshly ground black pepper

Using a vegetable peeler, peel carrots and cucumbers into long strips. Combine dressing ingredients in a jar and shake well to combine. Place sliced snow peas in a bowl and cover with boiling water. Stand for 1-2 minutes or until they turn bright green, then drain and rinse under cold water. Combine all of the vegetables in a bowl, drizzle with dressing and toss well to combine.

Nutrition information (per serve): kilojoules 280, calories 67, protein 3.5g, fat 2.5g, saturated fat 0.5g, carbohydrate 5.5g, fibre 3.5g.

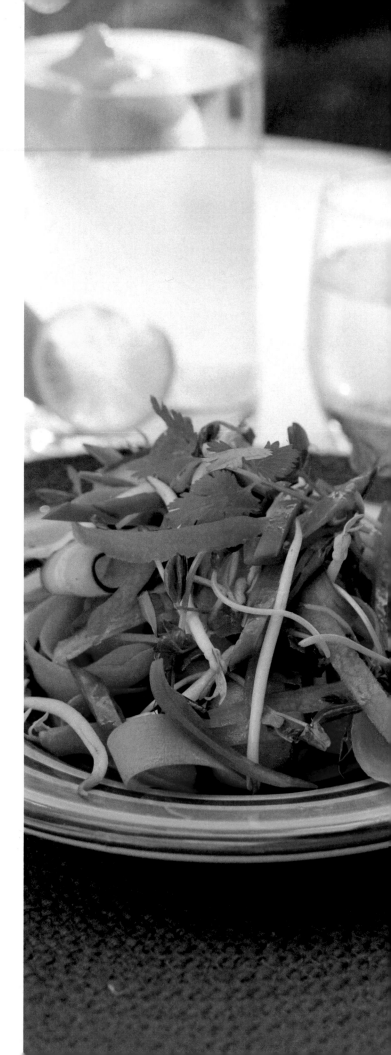

Mushroom Salad

Serves 4

5 cups mushrooms, sliced

1 red capsicum, finely diced

1 green capsicum, finely diced

½ red onion, finely diced

1 tablespoon parsley, chopped

¼ cup fat free French dressing

Freshly ground black pepper

Combine mushrooms, capsicums and red onion. Combine parsley, French dressing and pepper in a jar and shake well to combine. Drizzle dressing over vegetables and toss well to serve.

Nutrition information (per serve): kilojoules 235, calories 56, protein 4.5g, fat 0.5g, saturated fat negligible, carbohydrate 7g, fibre 3g.

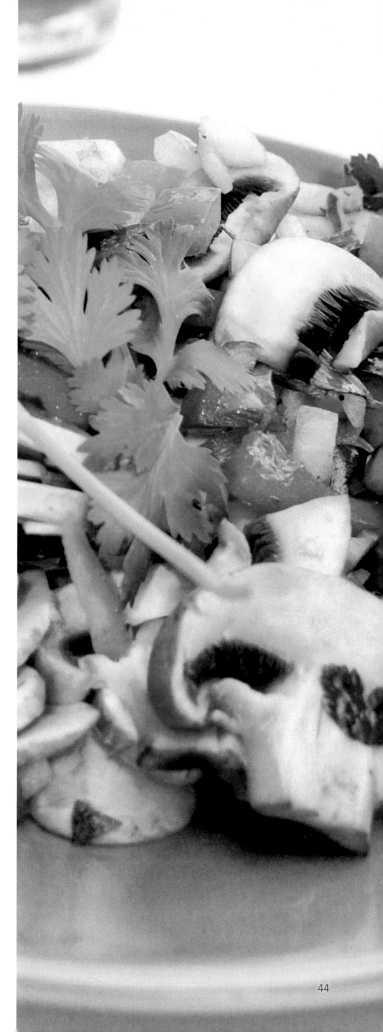

Vegetable Kebabs

Serves 4

1 tablespoon olive oil

1 clove garlic, crushed

¼ cup balsamic vinegar

1 zucchini, cut into 2cm chunks

4 yellow squash, cut into 2cm chunks

2 cups mushrooms, cut into 2cm chunks

1 red capsicum, cut into 3cm chunks

1 green capsicum, cut into 3cm chunks

1 red onion, cut into thin wedges

2 cups cherry tomatoes

Place all ingredients in a small plastic bag and seal. Shake and rub ingredients together until well combined. Thread vegetables onto skewers and reserve marinade. Place on grill over medium-hot heat. Baste occasionally with marinade. Grill 20 minutes or until tender.

Nutrition information (per serve): kilojoules 420, calories 100, protein 4g, fat 5g, saturated fat 0.5g, carbohydrate 7g, fibre 4.5g.

- Use metal skewers or soak wooden skewers in water prior to use to prevent burning.
- This recipe is useful if you are hosting or attending a barbeque whilst on a VLED program, enabling you to also enjoy the barbeque.

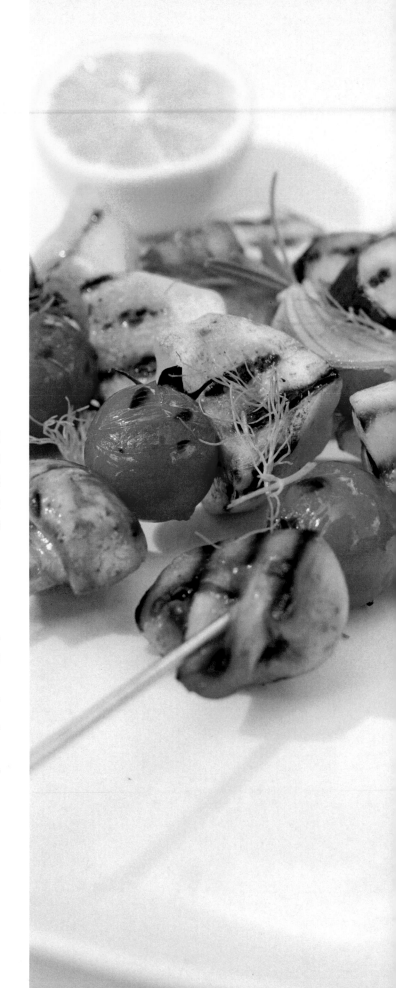

Cauliflower & Cabbage Curry

Serves 4

Oil spray

1 medium onion, chopped

1 cup salt reduced chicken stock

1 small head cauliflower (approx 4 cups), chopped into florets

½ cabbage, shredded

1 zucchini, diced

1 stick celery, diced

1 tablespoon curry powder (to taste)

Heat a frying pan that has been sprayed with oil. Add onion and cook until soft. Add stock and bring to the boil. Add cauliflower, zucchini, celery and curry powder, cover and cook for 5 minutes. Stir in cabbage, cover and cook for 5-10 minutes. Stir regularly. Simmer until sauce thickens.

Nutrition information (per serve): kilojoules 350, calories 84, protein 5g, fat 2g, saturated fat negligible, carbohydrate 8g, fibre 7.5g.

- This recipe is suitable to freeze.
- Enjoy curry with rice? Serve with konjac rice in place of normal rice whilst on the very low energy diet.

> **"Absolutely divine."**
> *- Debra, gastric band -*
>
> **"I fell in love with this, I lived on it!"**
> *- Barbara, gastric band -*
>
> **"We cooked some extra cauliflower in stock, pureed it and added to the curry to make it creamier. The boys enjoyed it too!"**
> *- Kym, gastric bypass -*

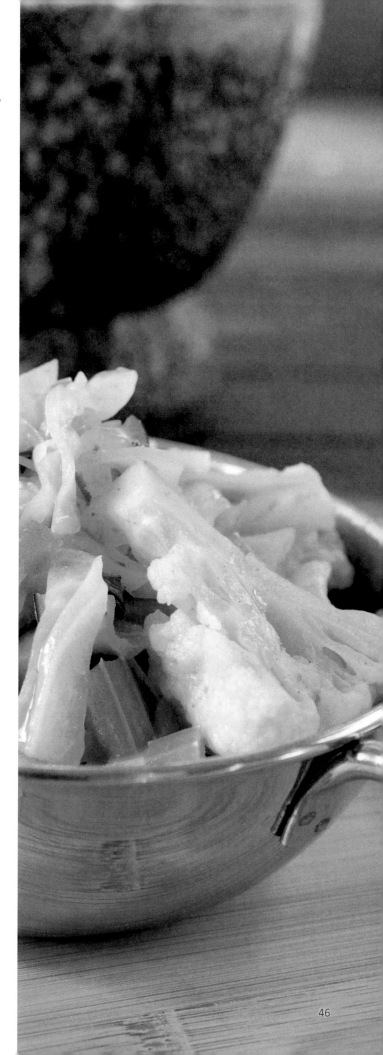

Spicy Vegetable Smoothie

Serves 4

3 cups no added salt tomato juice

1 red capsicum, roasted, peeled and diced

1 cucumber, peeled and chopped

1 tablespoon lemon or lime juice

¼ cup spring onions, chopped

1 tablespoon Worcestershire Sauce

Dash of Tabasco sauce

Freshly ground black pepper, to taste

Place all ingredients in a blender or food processor and puree until thin enough to drink through a thick straw.

Nutrition information (per cup): kilojoules 245, calories 59, protein 2.5g, fat negligible, saturated fat negligible, carbohydrate 8g, fibre 2g.

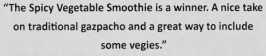

"The Spicy Vegetable Smoothie is a winner. A nice take on traditional gazpacho and a great way to include some vegies."
- *Robyn, gastric bypass* -

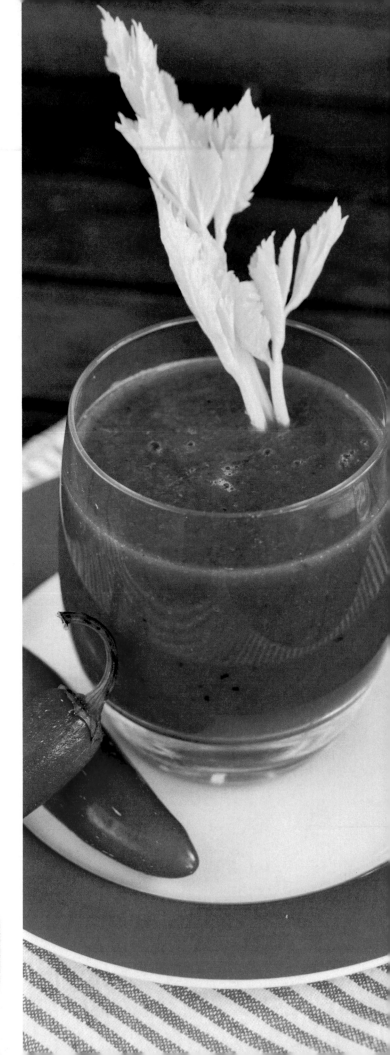

Balsamic Roasted Asparagus & Mushrooms

Serves 2

2 teaspoons olive oil

1 clove garlic, crushed

2 bunches of asparagus, ends trimmed

2 cups button mushrooms

2 tablespoons balsamic vinegar

Pinch of dried oregano

Freshly ground black pepper

Preheat oven to 220°C. Use a vegetable peeler to trim away some of the asparagus skin, in strips, from the stem ends of the spears. Place all ingredients in a small plastic bag and seal. Shake and rub ingredients together until well combined. Empty the contents of the bag on to a baking tray. Roast in the oven for 7 - 10 minutes until the vegetables are cooked to your liking.

Nutrition information (per serve): kilojoules 370, calories 89, protein 5.5g, fat 5g, saturated fat 0.5g, carbohydrate 3g, fibre 4g.

Capsicum and zucchini can replace the asparagus and mushrooms for variety. This recipe can also be cooked on a barbeque, which is useful if hosting or attending a social event whilst on the VLED program.

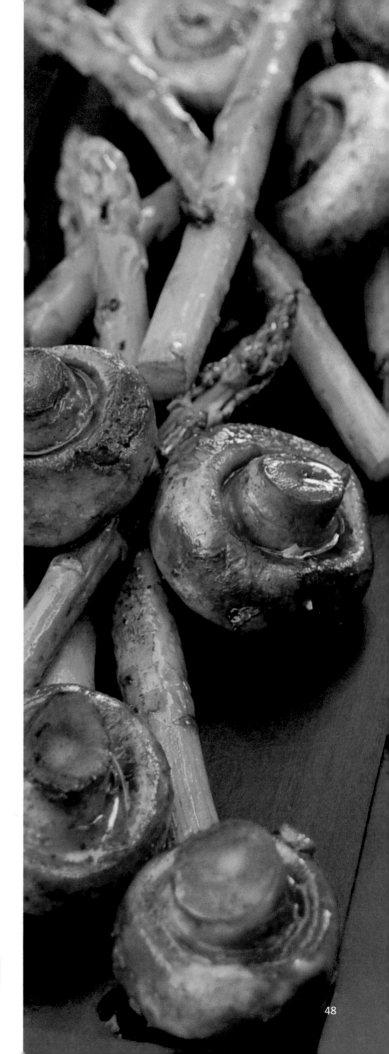

> **"That was nice."**
> *- Malcolm, gastric band -*

Lemon & Greens Smoothie

Serves 4

2 handfuls baby spinach

1 cucumber, chopped

2 sticks celery, strings removed and chopped

2 lemons, peeled and chopped

1 tablespoon fresh mint (or 1 teaspoon minced)

1 teaspoons minced ginger

1 cup water

2 cups ice cubes

Combine all ingredients in a blender or food processor and puree until smooth.

Nutrition information (per serve): kilojoules 95, calories 23, protein 1g, fat negligible, saturated fat nil, carbohydrate 2.5g, fibre 2g.

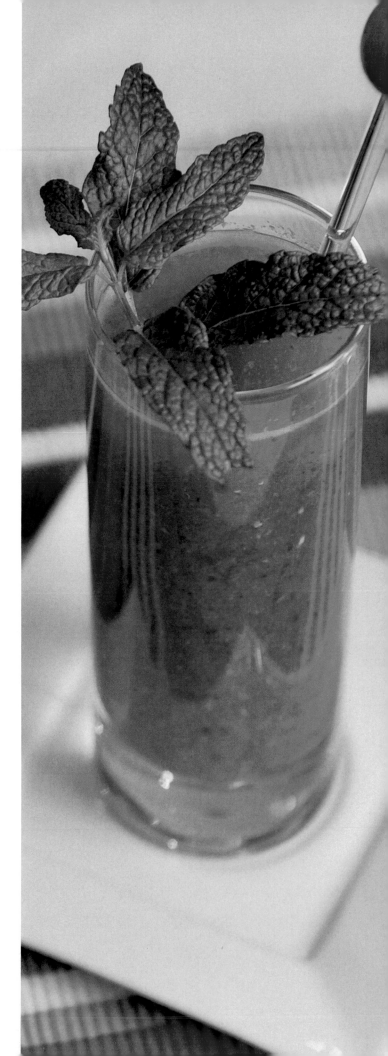

Broccoli with Fennel

Serves 4

Oil spray

1 teaspoon fennel seeds

1 bulb fennel, diced

1 onion, finely diced

1 large head broccoli (or 2 small heads), trimmed

A sprinkle of thyme and basil

⅔ cup salt reduced chicken stock

Heat a large frying pan that has been sprayed with oil. Add the fennel seeds and stir. Cook for a few minutes. Whilst the fennel seeds cook, chop the fennel bulb and onion. Add the fennel to the frying pan as it is ready, followed by the onion. Cook until soft, a few minutes. While the fennel and onion cooks, trim the broccoli. Add the broccoli, herbs and stock to the frying pan and stir to slightly coat the broccoli with liquid. Cover and let cook for 5 minutes. Uncover, stir and cover again, turn off the heat and let rest, covered, for another 5 minutes.

Nutrition information (per serve): kilojoules 350, calories 84, protein 8g, fat 2g, saturated fat negligible, carbohydrate 4.5g, fibre 8g.

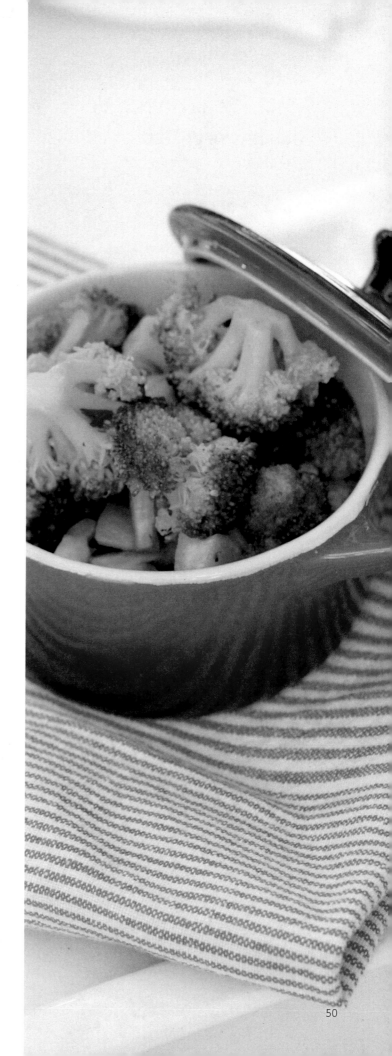

Snack Ideas on the Very Low Energy Diet

Cauliflower Popcorn

Oil spray

Cauliflower

Herb or spice of your choice eg. turmeric, cumin, chilli powder, curry powder, garlic powder, black pepper

Preheat oven to 200°C. Break cauliflower into popcorn-like, bite-size florets. Spread over a baking tray lined with baking paper. Spray with oil spray, then sprinkle lightly with herb/s or spice/s of your choice. Bake 20 to 30 minutes or until the cauliflower is slightly browned. Serve.

Kale Chips

Olive oil spray

Bunch of kale

Dried chilli

Garlic powder

Preheat oven to 160°C. Spread kale over a baking tray lined with baking paper. Spray with oil spray, then sprinkle lightly with chilli and garlic powder. Bake for approximately 10 minutes. Watch closely to ensure kale does not burn. Serve.

Recipe suggestion courtesy of Bianca, gastric bypass, 2013.

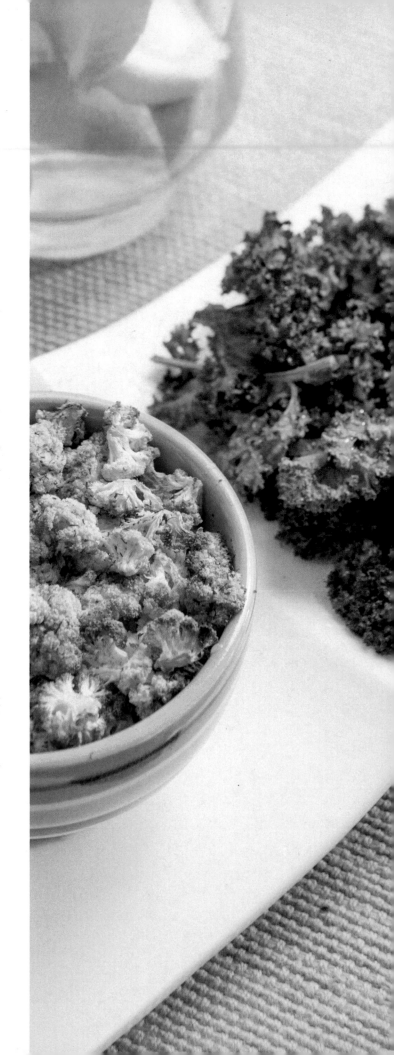

Recovering from Surgery: Fluid, Smooth Pureed and Soft Diets

Fluid Diet

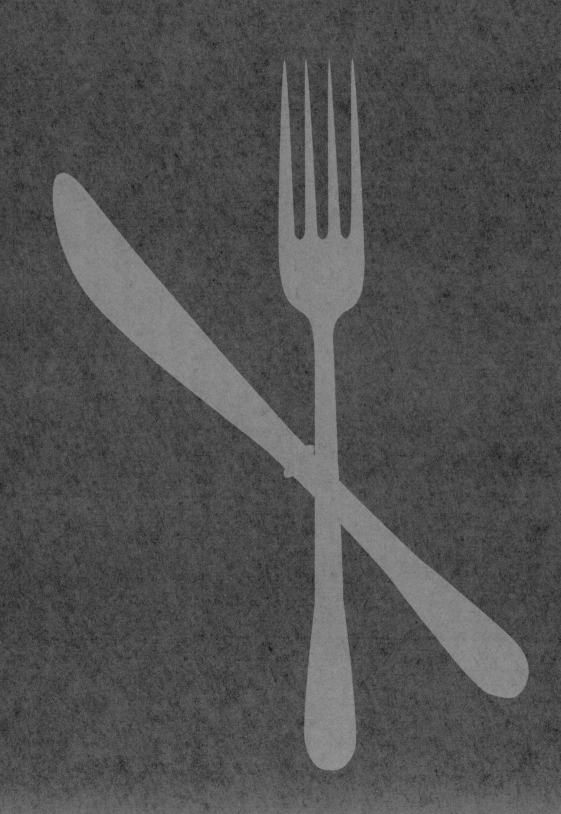

Recovery Stage 1: Fluid Diet

As described earlier, all forms of weight loss surgery will cause some swelling of the digestive tract. You must remain on a fluid diet to allow any stitching to heal and the swelling to subside.

Immediately after surgery, drink small amounts slowly, such as 50ml per hour. Drinking large amounts may cause pain, discomfort or vomiting. Vomiting must be avoided.

When your first meal tray of fluid arrives in hospital, do not drink all fluids at once. Sip slowly and spread fluid out over the day. To sip slowly, imagine each drink is a steaming hot cup of tea or coffee. If you tend to drink large amounts quickly or 'gulp' your fluids, use a medicine cup (50ml) and drink from this until you adapt to drinking smaller amounts.

In hospital you may be required to have clear fluid initially. You will be advised when you can progress to a broader range of fluids.

On the fluid diet, suitable fluids are those thin enough to pass through a straw.

Just because food is sent to you on your tray in hospital does not mean you should eat it. A hospital kitchen is a busy place and mistakes can occur. If solid food is delivered to you, don't eat it. Remind hospital staff that you need fluid that is thin enough to pass through a straw.

Remain on the fluid diet for as long as your surgical team recommends.

The different types of surgery have a different effect on the stomach. Depending on the surgery you have had, your surgeon's technique and your individual recovery, he or she will have specific recommendations for the time required to stay on a fluid diet after surgery.

A *Fluid Diet Sample Menu* is provided (page 57) and our surgical team recommend you stay on this for two weeks. This is a suggestion only. If your support team recommends differently, follow their advice.

Protein on the fluid diet

Protein is used to build and repair and will help the body heal after surgery. Normally when we think of protein foods we think of meat, chicken, fish and eggs. When on a fluid diet you will need different sources of protein. Protein from milk is the most common fluid source. Where possible, it is best to meet your protein target with whole or 'normal' food or drink, however, it can be very difficult to reach your protein targets in the early stages following surgery when on the fluid or smooth puree diet.

There are a range of commercially available protein supplements that you can add to fluids to boost your protein intake on the fluid diet. When choosing a protein supplement, look for those based on whey protein isolate as these are rapidly absorbed by the body.

Whilst most commercially available protein supplements offer a milky type product, one Australian company has developed some clear, whey protein isolate products. BODIE'z clear protein waters and powders are a great way of increasing your protein intake without the milky taste or texture. You can find out more about BODIE'z clear protein waters at www.bodiezpro.com. When placing an order be sure to use our Nutrition for Weight Loss Surgery discount code, NFWLS.

The Smoothies & Soups (from page 58) are good

sources of protein and additional protein powder can be added if desired.

Fluids low in protein can be sipped between meals to keep you hydrated.

Everyone will recover differently after surgery, therefore some people will tolerate a greater amount of fluid than others. Those with a gastric band will tend to tolerate a greater volume than those with a sleeve or gastric bypass.

The sample menu over the page is just an example of how you could plan your fluid intake over the day. The key is to sip slowly and stop as soon as you feel satisfied. You do not want to drink to the point of discomfort.

Try to include six, small fluid meals daily and choose higher protein options where possible.

Best Choices: Fluids High in Protein (choose for meals)

- *Smoothies & Soups* (from page 58)
- Home made smoothies, milkshakes or milk coffees, made with low or reduced fat milk with added protein powder (look for whey protein isolate powders).
- Home made smoothies, milkshakes or milk coffees made with high protein milk (such as The Complete Dairy™ milks).
- VLED milkshakes or soups such as Optifast® VLCD, KicStart® VLCD or Dr. MacLeod's®, which are high in vitamins and minerals, hence a good choice on the fluid diet.
- BODIE'z berry or kiwi clear protein water (available at www.bodiezpro.com and you can use our discount code, NFWLS).
- Home made soup made with beef, chicken, fish or legumes, pureed until it is thin enough to get through a straw. Add whey protein isolate powder as desired.

Include Less Often: Fluids Low in Protein (drink between meals)

- water
- tea
- herbal tea
- coffee
- vegetable juice
- diet cordials
- canned soups

FLUID DIET SAMPLE MENU

Breakfast Options

- VLED milkshake
- Lemon Smoothie (page 59)
- Choc Coconut Smoothie (page 60)
- Strawberry Whip (page 61)
- Banana & Cinnamon Smoothie (page 62)
- Blueberry Smoothie (page 63)
- Carrot & Apple Smoothie (page 64)
- Home made smoothie or milkshake or milk coffee made with low or reduced fat milk with added whey protein isolate powder
- Home made smoothie, milkshake or milk coffee made with high protein milk such as The Complete Dairy™ milk.

Lunch Options

- VLED milkshake or soup
- Beetroot, Walnut & Feta Smoothie (page 65)
- Sweet Potato Soup (page 66)
- Chicken & Artichoke Soup (page 67)
- Tomato Beef Soup (page 68)
- Creamy Prawn Soup (page 69)
- Cauliflower & Ham Soup (page 70)
- Curried Pumpkin & Lentil Soup (page 71)
- Mexican Beef Soup (page 72)
- Zucchini, Pea & Bacon Soup (page 73)
- Home made soup made with beef, chicken, fish or legumes, pureed until it is thin enough to get through a straw. Add whey protein isolate powder as desired.

Dinner Options

As per lunch suggestions.

Mid Morning, Mid Afternoon and Supper

Sip on any of the suggested smoothies, milk based coffee, VLED milkshakes or BODIE'z protein water* as tolerated.

BODIE'z clear protein waters are available at www.bodiezpro.com. When placing an order be sure to use our Nutrition for Weight Loss Surgery discount code, NFWLS.

Using the Smoothie and Soup Recipes

Serving sizes

The smoothie and soup recipes are designed to make approximately four, one cup serves, or approximately one litre in total.

Immediately following sleeve gastrectomy or gastric bypass surgery, you may only tolerate one quarter to half a cup at a time.

Immediately following gastric band surgery, you may tolerate half a cup at one time. As your swelling subsides, some may tolerate one cup. Everyone recovers differently and will tolerate different amounts. Sip slowly and stop before you feel any discomfort.

If you only tolerate smaller amounts, make sure you include VLED products (such as Optifast VLCD®, KicStart® VLCD or Dr. MacLeod's®) and higher protein soups and smoothies. See the nutrition information provided with each recipe to choose the higher protein options. You can also use whey protein isolate powders to add additional protein to your fluids and sip on BODIE'z clear protein waters throughout the day.

All smoothie and soup recipes are suitable to freeze, or to share with family and friends. Use small freezer bags or containers to freeze in single serves if you only tolerate small amounts. Smoothies also freeze well to make ice blocks, which may help increase your intake if you are struggling to obtain adequate fluid.

Please note that once you have recovered fully from surgery, pureed fluids are not likely to be as satisfying as solid foods, hence pureed soups should be used during recovery only.

Ingredients

Many of the soup recipes used on the fluid diet include stock as an ingredient. If using commercial stocks, choose the salt reduced varieties. Alternatively, the *Ingredients* pages at the end of the *Recipes for Healthy Living* section provide recipes for producing stocks from scratch (page 214). These will provide a flavoursome stock without the salt of the commercial varieties.

The *Ingredients* pages at the end of the *Recipes for Healthy Living* section provide recipes for cooking legumes from the dried form (page 212). This provides an alternative to using the tinned varieties. If you choose to use the tinned legumes, drain and rinse well.

Hints and tips

Throughout the recipes, practical hints and tips are included between the yellow lines.

> "Thanks so much for saving me from the tyranny of the dreaded shakes! I still remember the fantastic feeling when I had the Beetroot, Walnut and Feta Smoothie after 10 days of Optifast and then clear fluids. I thought I'd died and gone to heaven!"
>
> *- Kerry, gastric band -*
>
> "As someone who has undergone gastric bypass surgery, all of the smoothie recipes worked really well following surgery. They were delicious, easy to digest and flavoursome."
>
> *- Robyn, gastric bypass -*
>
> "The soups were really handy as I didn't have much idea of what to put in there".
>
> *- Jenny, gastric band -*
>
> "I had my gastric sleeve in January 2011 and I don't know where I'd be without your book. Post op, the soups have been invaluable."
>
> *- Kate, sleeve gastrectomy -*

Lemon Smoothie

Makes 4 cups

2 cups low or reduced fat milk

1 cup Chobani® lemon or vanilla yoghurt

Juice and rind of 1 lemon

2 tablespoons (30g) whey protein isolate powder

Dissolve protein powder in half a cup of the milk. Place all ingredients, except the milk containing the protein powder in a blender or food processor and blend until well combined. Slowly add the dissolved powder and blend on low speed until combined.

Nutrition information (per cup): kilojoules 630, calories 150, protein 18g, fat 1.5g, saturated fat 1g, carbohydrate 6.5g, fibre negligible.

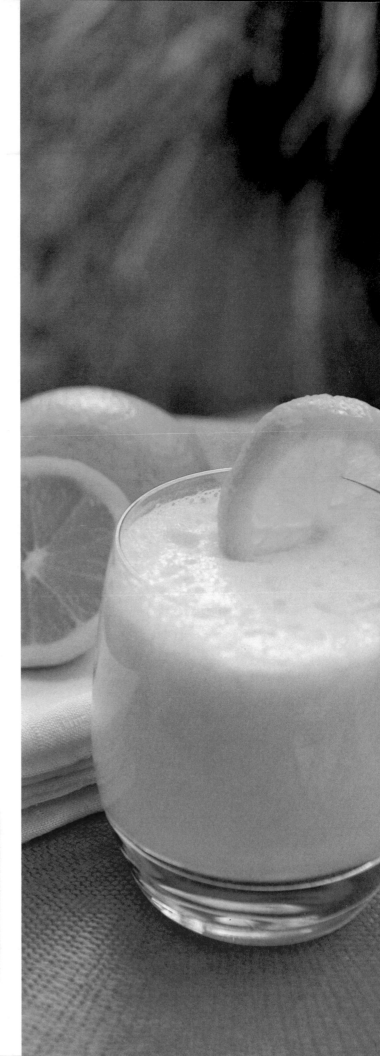

> **"The Lemon Smoothie is my favourite."**
> *- Jo, gastric band -*
>
> **"This was incredible, reminded me of lemon cheesecake!"**
> *- Sam, gastric band -*
>
> **"I used lime instead of lemon as I have a lime tree - that was really nice."**
> *- Helen, gastric band -*

Choc Coconut Smoothie

Makes 4 cups

2 cups low or reduced fat milk

1½ cups Chobani® coconut yoghurt

¼ teaspoon coconut essence

1 tablespoon cocoa

2 tablespoons (30g) whey protein isolate powder

Dissolve protein powder in half a cup of the milk. Place all ingredients, except the milk containing the protein powder in a blender or food processor and blend until well combined. Slowly add the dissolved powder and blend on low speed to combine.

Nutrition information (per cup): kilojoules 750, calories 179, protein 19g, fat 3.5g, saturated fat 2g, carbohydrate 18g, fibre 0.5g.

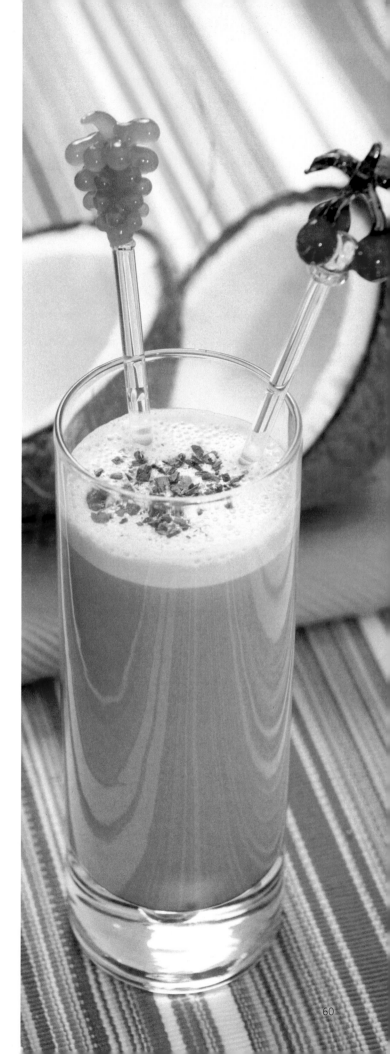

Strawberry Whip

Makes 4 cups

1 cup strawberries, tops removed

1 cup low or reduced fat milk

1 tub (170g) Chobani® strawberry yoghurt

½ cup apple and blackcurrant juice

3 tablespoons (45g) whey protein isolate powder

Dissolve protein powder in half a cup of the milk. Place all ingredients, except the milk containing the protein powder in a blender or food processor and puree until thin enough to drink through a thick straw. Slowly add the dissolved powder and blend until combined.

Nutrition information (per cup): kilojoules 540, calories 129, protein 16.5g, fat 1g, saturated fat 0.5g, carbohydrate 13g, fibre negligible.

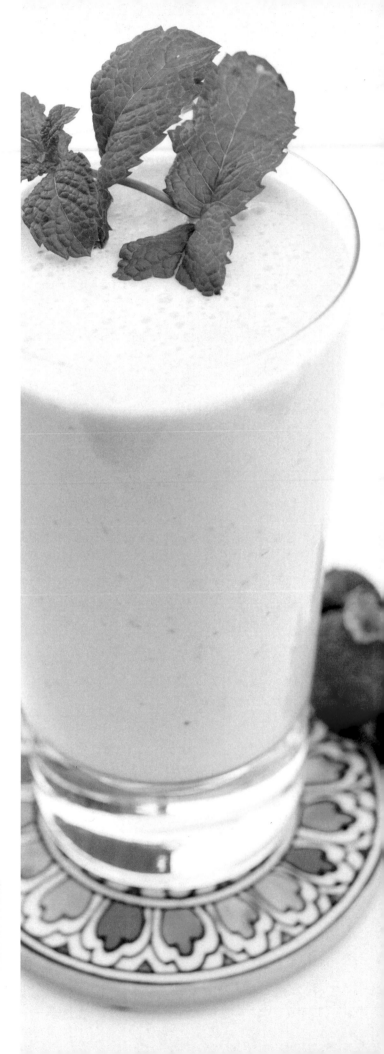

> **"Really nice."**
> *- Karina, sleeve gastrectomy -*
>
> **"I'm not a huge fan of berries, but really enjoyed this. I like the tangy flavour."**
> *- Amy, gastric band -*

Banana Cinnamon Smoothie

Makes 4 cups

2 small ripe bananas, chopped

1½ cups low or reduced fat milk

1 tub (170g) or 2/3 cup Chobani® vanilla yoghurt

3 tablespoons (45g) whey protein isolate powder

Sprinkle of cinnamon

Dissolve protein powder in half a cup of the milk. Place all ingredients, except the milk containing the protein powder in a blender or food processor and puree until thin enough to drink through a thick straw. Slowly add the dissolved powder and blend on low speed to combine. Pour into a glass and sprinkle with cinnamon.

Nutrition information (per cup): kilojoules 705, calories 169, protein 18g, fat 2g, saturated fat 1g, carbohydrate 19.5g, fibre 1g.

A teaspoon of cocoa instead of cinnamon makes a tasty choc-banana variation.

"The Banana & Cinnamon Smoothie is delicious and the yoghurt gives the drink an appealing creamy texture."
- Robyn, gastric bypass -

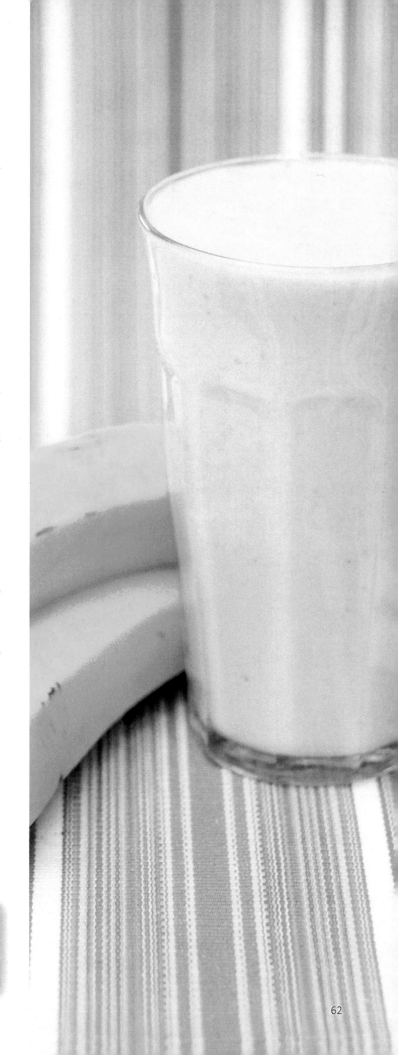

Blueberry Smoothie

Makes 4 cups

1 cup of chilled fresh or frozen blueberries, slightly thawed

1 cup milk

1 tub (170g) Chobani® blueberry yoghurt

3 tablespoons (45g) whey protein isolate powder

Dissolve protein powder in half a cup of the milk. Place all ingredients, except the milk containing the protein powder in a blender or food processor and puree until thin enough to drink through a thick straw. Slowly add the dissolved powder and blend on low speed to combine.

Nutrition information (per cup): kilojoules 535, calories 128, protein 16g, fat 1g, saturated fat 0.5g, carbohydrate 13.5g, fibre negligible.

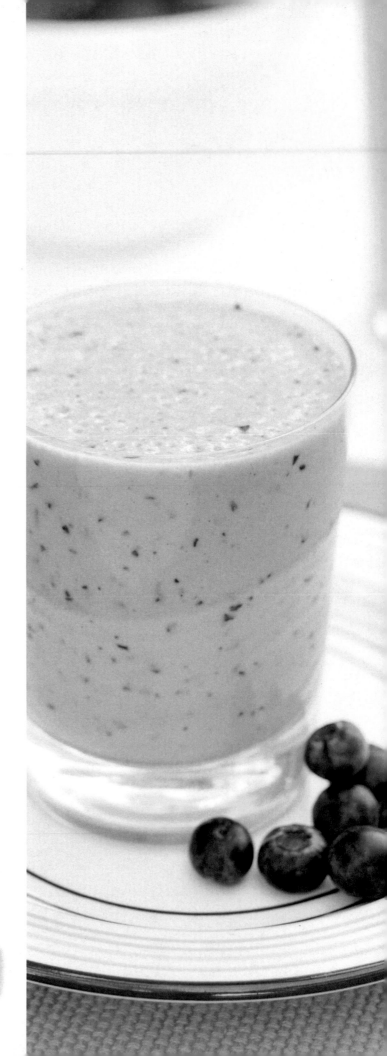

"This was really good!"

- Danielle, gastric band -

Carrot & Apple Smoothie

Makes 4 cups

3 carrots, peeled and chopped

1 cup canned pie apple

1 cup low or reduced fat milk

½ cup Chobani® plain low fat yoghurt

3 tablespoons (45g) whey protein isolate powder

Dissolve protein powder in half a cup of the milk. Place carrots in saucepan and cover with water. Bring to the boil and simmer until soft. Allow to cool, then add to a blender or food processor with the pie apple and yoghurt. Puree until thin enough to drink through a thick straw. Slowly add the dissolved powder and blend on low speed to combine.

Nutrition information (per cup): kilojoules 575, calories 138, protein 16g, fat 1.5g, saturated fat 1g, carbohydrate 14g, fibre 2.5g.

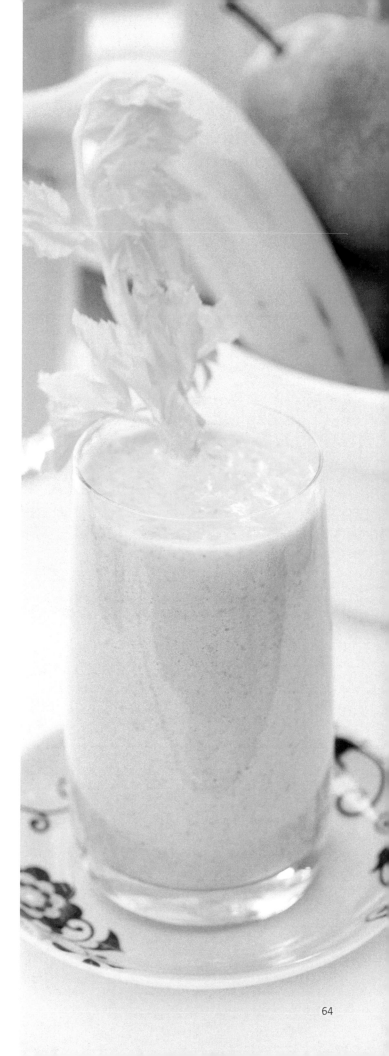

Beetroot, Walnut & Feta Smoothie

Makes 4 cups

450g can diced beetroot

100g low fat feta cheese

½ cup canned pie apple

¼ cup walnuts, finely chopped

170g Chobani® plain low fat yoghurt

2 tablespoons (30g) whey protein isolate powder

½ cup water

Dissolve protein powder in water. Place beetroot, including the fluid from the can, in a blender or food processor. Add feta and blend until smooth. Add canned apple, walnuts and yoghurt and puree until thin enough to drink through a thick straw. Slowly add the dissolved powder and blend on low speed to combine.

Nutrition information (per cup): kilojoules 940, calories 225, protein 20g, fat 10g, saturated fat 3g, carbohydrate 12g, fibre 4.5g.

> "I particularly like the Lemon Smoothie and the Beetroot, Walnut and Feta."
>
> *- Kerry, gastric band -*
>
> "Beautiful!"
>
> *- Sarah, gastric band -*

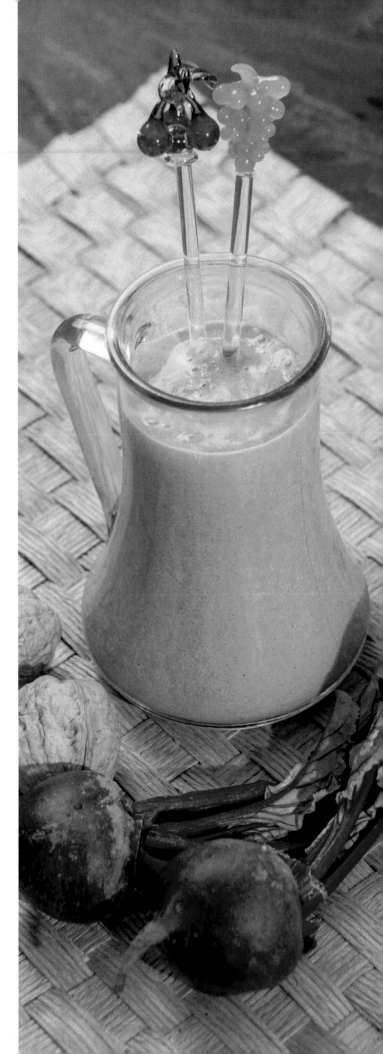

Sweet Potato Soup

Makes 4 cups

Oil spray

2 cups sweet potato, diced

2 cups salt reduced chicken or vegetable stock

½ onion, diced

1 clove garlic, crushed

⅓ cup zucchini, grated

¼ cup red lentils, washed

⅓ cup capsicum, roasted, rinsed and diced

½ cup low fat milk

1 tablespoon lemon juice

3 tablespoons (45g) whey protein isolate powder

Heat a large saucepan that has been sprayed with oil. Add onion and garlic and cook gently. Add sweet potato, zucchini, lentils and stock and simmer until the lentils are soft. Add the capsicum and remove from heat. Leave to cool slightly. Dissolve protein powder in milk. Pour soup into a blender or food processor and puree. Whilst pureeing, slowly add the milk mixture and lemon juice and continue to puree until soup is thin enough to drink through a thick straw. Return to saucepan and reheat gently to serve, but do not boil.

Nutrition information (per cup): kilojoules 700, calories 167, protein 16.5g, fat 2g, saturated fat 0.5g, carbohydrate 19g, fibre 3.5g.

> "I added leek and pumpkin - wow, that was good!"
> - Simon, gastric band -

> "The Sweet Potato Soup, that was my absolute favourite!"
> - Tania, gastric bypass -

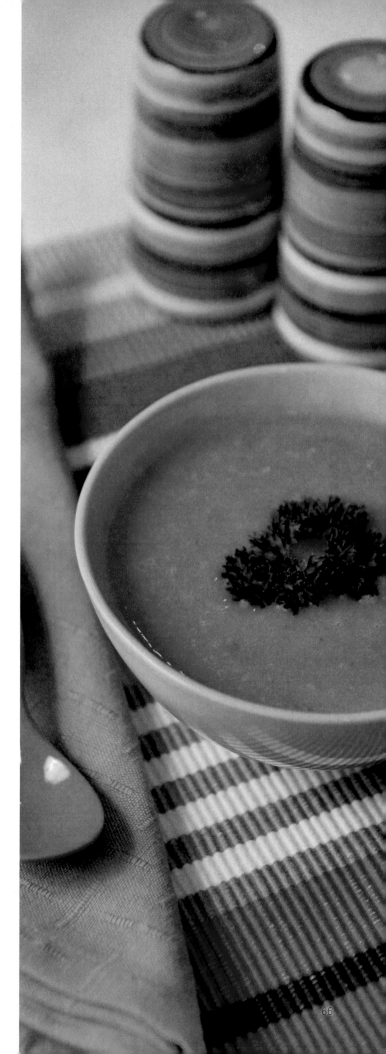

Chicken & Artichoke Soup

Makes 4 cups

400g can artichoke hearts, rinsed and drained

2 tablespoons grated Parmesan cheese

2 tablespoons lemon juice

2 teaspoons lemon zest

1 teaspoon dried tarragon

2 cloves garlic, crushed

¼ teaspoon ground nutmeg

¼ teaspoon chilli powder

2 cups salt reduced chicken stock

300g skinless chicken, trimmed of fat eg. breast, thigh, or tenderloin

185ml low fat evaporated milk

Puree artichoke hearts in a food processor until smooth. Add lemon juice, lemon zest, tarragon, garlic, nutmeg, chilli powder and stock to a large saucepan and bring to the boil. Once boiling, place the chicken into the stock and simmer gently for 15-20 minutes until chicken is cooked through. Remove the chicken and dice. Pour the stock into a blender or food processor with the artichokes, chicken and parmesan cheese and puree. Whilst pureeing, slowly add the evaporated milk and continue to puree until soup is thin enough to drink through a thick straw. Pour into saucepan and reheat gently to serve, but do not boil.

Nutrition information (per cup): kilojoules 775, calories 185, protein 23g, fat 6.5g, saturated fat 3g, carbohydrate 7g, fibre 2g.

For a Middle Eastern flavour variation, add ¼ teaspoon ground cumin, ½ teaspoon cinnamon and ½ teaspoon turmeric to the stock, and 50g low fat feta cheese instead of Parmesan.

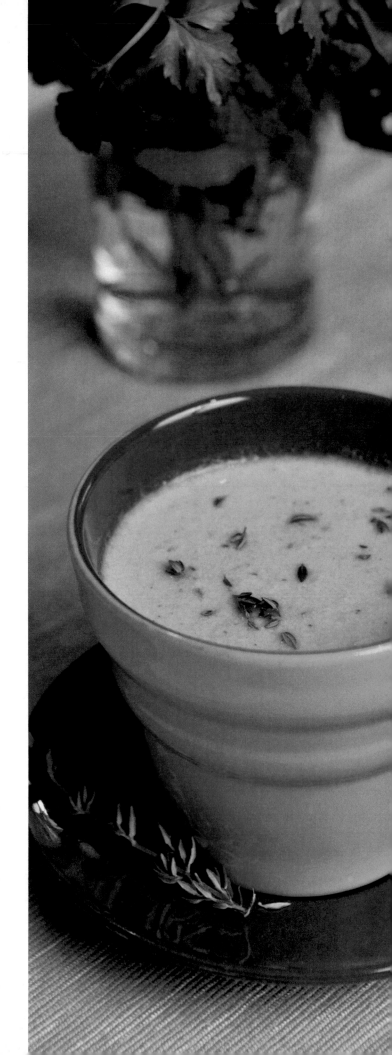

Tomato Beef Soup

Makes 4 cups

Oil spray

250g lean mince eg. premium or extra trim

1 onion, diced

1 stick celery, finely diced

1 clove garlic, crushed

1 bay leaf

½ teaspoon dried basil

1½ cups no added salt tomato juice

¼ cup cooked red kidney beans

1 carrot, diced

1 cup salt reduced vegetable stock

Heat a large saucepan that has been sprayed with oil. Brown mince, onion, garlic and celery, breaking the mince into small pieces whilst cooking. Add the remaining ingredients and bring to the boil. Cover and simmer gently until carrot is tender. Puree soup in blender or food processor until soup is thin enough to drink through a thick straw. Return to saucepan and reheat to serve.

Nutrition information (per cup): kilojoules 610, calories 146, protein 15g, fat 6g, saturated fat 2g, carbohydrate 6g, fibre 2.5g.

Don't have time to be cooking separate meals for family or friends? Set aside your serves, then mix this soup through some cooked pasta for the family. Fold in some baby spinach and sprinkle with parmesan cheese.

> "I had a crack at the Tomato Beef Soup. It was nice and actually a bit of fun making it."
> - Brett, sleeve gastrectomy -

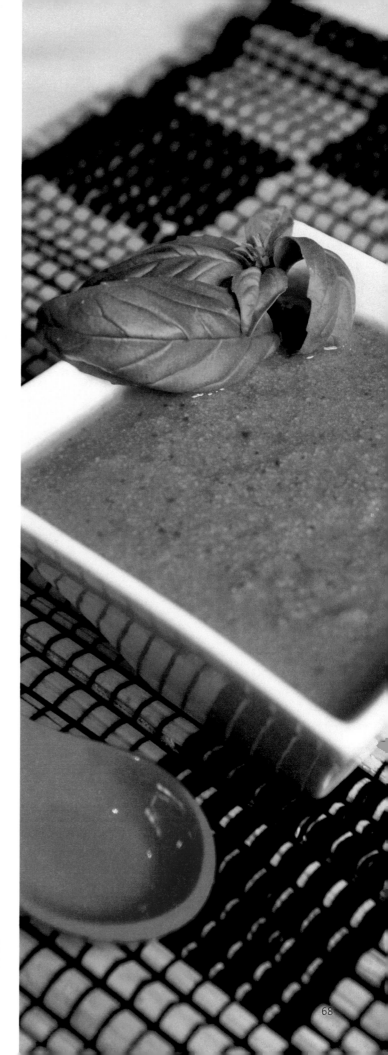

Creamy Prawn Soup

Makes 4 cups

Oil spray

2 tablespoons grated onion

¼ stick celery, finely diced

¼ cup zucchini, grated

2 teaspoons plain flour

1 cup warm low fat milk

2 tablespoons roasted capsicum, rinsed and diced

1 tablespoon tomato paste

1 teaspoon lemon zest, finely grated

2 teaspoons lemon juice

2 teaspoons chives, chopped

2 teaspoons parsley, chopped

Pinch of nutmeg

375ml can low fat evaporated milk

300g green prawn meat

Freshly ground black pepper

Heat a saucepan that has been sprayed with oil. Add onion, celery and zucchini and cook gently for 2 minutes. Stir in flour, then warm milk. Add tomato paste, roasted capsicum, lemon zest, lemon juice, chives, parsley, nutmeg and evaporated milk. Heat through until hot, but not boiling. Add the prawn meat and cook gently for 2-3 minutes until the prawns have changed colour. Remove from heat and leave to cool slightly before pouring into a blender or food processor. Puree soup until it is thin enough to drink through a thick straw. Return to saucepan and reheat gently to serve, but do not boil.

Nutrition information (per cup): kilojoules 900, calories 215, protein 27g, fat 4g, saturated fat 1.5g, carbohydrate 17.5g, fibre 1g.

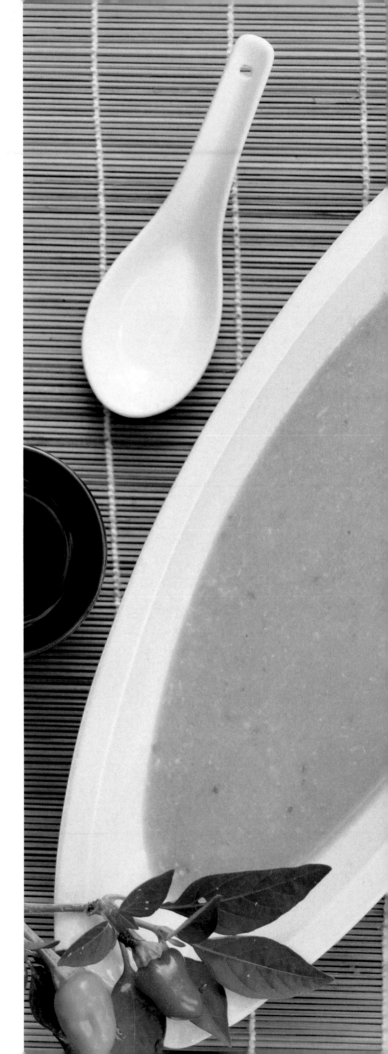

Cauliflower & Ham Soup

Makes 4 cups

Oil spray

½ onion, diced

1 small or ½ large carrot, peeled and diced

3 sprigs parsley, chopped

3 cups of cauliflower florets

¼ cup zucchini, finely diced

100g lean ham, diced

1 tablespoon chopped, fresh basil

1½ cups salt reduced vegetable stock

375ml can low fat evaporated milk

Heat a large saucepan that has been sprayed with oil. Add carrot, zucchini and onion. Cook, covered for a few minutes over a gentle heat with 1 tablespoon of stock to allow the flavours to develop. Add parsley, cauliflower, ham and basil. Stir well, then add the stock and bring to the boil. Reduce heat to a gentle simmer, and cook, covered until vegetables are very tender, about 30 minutes.

Remove soup from heat and leave to cool slightly. Once cool, pour soup into a blender or food processor. Whilst pureeing, slowly pour in the milk. Puree until the soup is thin enough to drink through a thick straw. Return to saucepan and reheat to serve, but do not boil.

Nutrition information (per cup): kilojoules 710, calories 170, protein 15g, fat 5g, saturated fat 2g, carbohydrate 15g, fibre 2g.

Assume all creamy soups are high in fat? Not when the creamy taste comes from low fat evaporated milk.

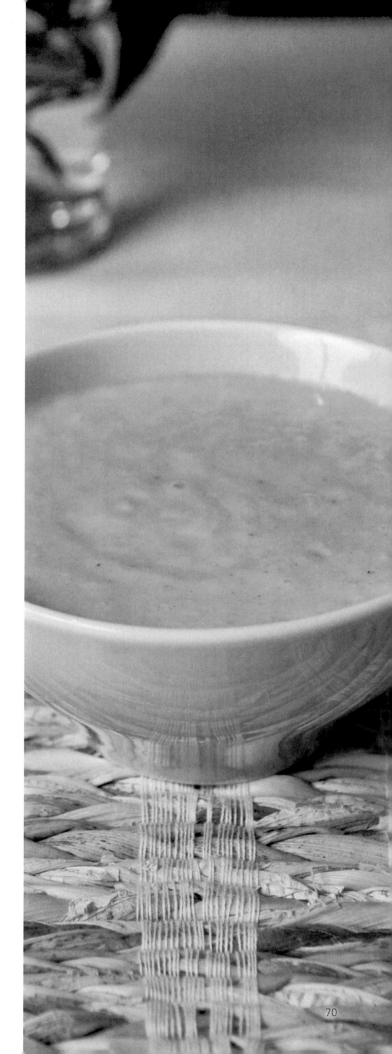

Curried Pumpkin & Lentil Soup

Makes 4 cups

1 onion, diced

1½ cups salt reduced chicken stock

1-2 teaspoons curry powder, to taste

3 cups pumpkin, diced

⅓ cup red lentils, washed

½ cup low fat evaporated milk

2 tablespoons (30g) whey protein isolate powder

½ cup Chobani® plain low fat yoghurt

2 tablespoons smooth peanut butter

Place first 5 ingredients into a large saucepan. Bring to the boil, cover and simmer gently until pumpkin is cooked and the lentils are tender, approximately 30-45 minutes. Remove from heat and leave to cool slightly. Pour pumpkin mixture into a blender or food processor and puree. Dissolve protein powder in milk. Whilst pureeing, slowly add the yoghurt and milk mixture and continue to puree until soup is thin enough to drink through a thick straw. Return to the saucepan and stir peanut butter through whilst re-heating, but do not boil.

Nutrition information (per cup): kilojoules 1030, calories 246, protein 22g, fat 8.5g, saturated fat 2g, carbohydrate 19g, fibre 5g.

> **"This was my favourite. I added roasted capsicum and that really made it."**
> *- Danielle, gastric band -*
>
> **"Beautiful, I absolutely love making this one."**
> *- Evelyn, gastric band -*
>
> **"Wholesome, very flavoursome."**
> *- Tiffany, gastric band -*
>
> **"This is beautiful. Hubby loves it too. The peanut butter adds a satay flavour."**
> *- Natalie, gastric band -*

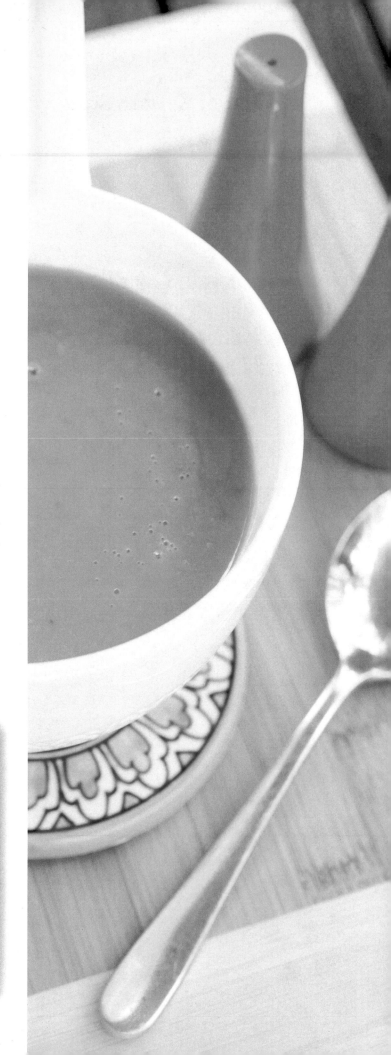

Mexican Beef Soup

Makes 4 cups

Oil spray

½ red onion, diced

200g beef, trimmed of fat, diced

35g packet salt reduced taco seasoning

2 cups water

400g no added salt, chopped tinned tomatoes

1 tablespoon no added salt tomato paste

¼ cup red kidney beans, rinsed and drained

⅓ cup fresh coriander leaves

4 tablespoons Chobani® plain low fat yoghurt

Heat a saucepan that has been sprayed with oil. Add the onion and cook, stirring, until soft. Add the beef and cook until the beef is starting to brown. Add the taco seasoning and cook, stirring, for 1-2 minutes. Add the water, tomatoes and tomato paste and bring to the boil. Reduce heat to low and simmer, covered, until the beef is cooked, approximately 40 minutes. Add the beans and coriander to the soup and cook, stirring occasionally, for 5 minutes or until heated through. Remove from heat and leave to cool slightly. Pour soup into a blender or food processor and puree until soup is thin enough to drink through a thick straw. Serve with a tablespoon of natural yoghurt.

Nutrition information (per cup): kilojoules 625, calories 149, protein 15g, fat 4.5g, saturated fat 1.5g, carbohydrate 10.5g, fibre 3g.

> **"My first home cooked meal after gastric bypass was the Mexican Beef Soup. It was yummo! My first taste of meat after surgery - I love my meat."**
> *- Courtney, gastric bypass -*
>
> **"Food highlight post op: Mexican Beef Soup from Sally's book."**
> *- Ben, gastric band -*

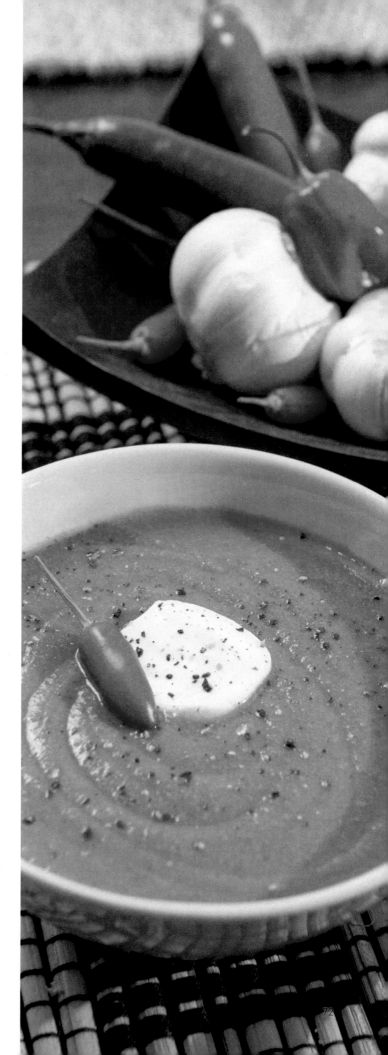

Zucchini, Pea & Bacon Soup

Makes 4 cups

Oil spray

1 onion, diced

1 garlic clove, crushed

175g short cut bacon, trimmed and chopped (approx 135g once trimmed)

2 cups zucchini, diced

1 cup frozen peas

2 cups salt reduced vegetable stock

1 tablespoon parmesan cheese

Freshly ground black pepper

2 tablespoons (35g) whey protein isolate powder

Heat a saucepan that has been sprayed with oil. Add onion, garlic and bacon, and cook, stirring, for 10 minutes. Add zucchini, peas and stock and bring to the boil. Reduce heat and simmer, covered, for 20 minutes or until zucchini is tender. Remove from heat and leave to cool slightly. Add parmesan cheese and season with black pepper. Pour soup into a blender or food processor and puree until soup is thin enough to drink through a thick straw. Dissolve protein powder in one quarter of a cup of water and stir through soup.

Nutrition information (per cup): kilojoules 705, calories 169, protein 18.5g, fat 6g, saturated fat 2g, carbohydrate 8g, fibre 4g.

> "I thought I was making this for myself but it was soon gone as the whole family loved it. They had theirs with a crumpet. It was satisfying and tasty and we all enjoyed it. I will be doing this one again."
> - *Gayleen, gastric bypass -*

> "We've tried every soup recipe. I'm now giving them to all my friends."
> - *Graham, gastric band -*

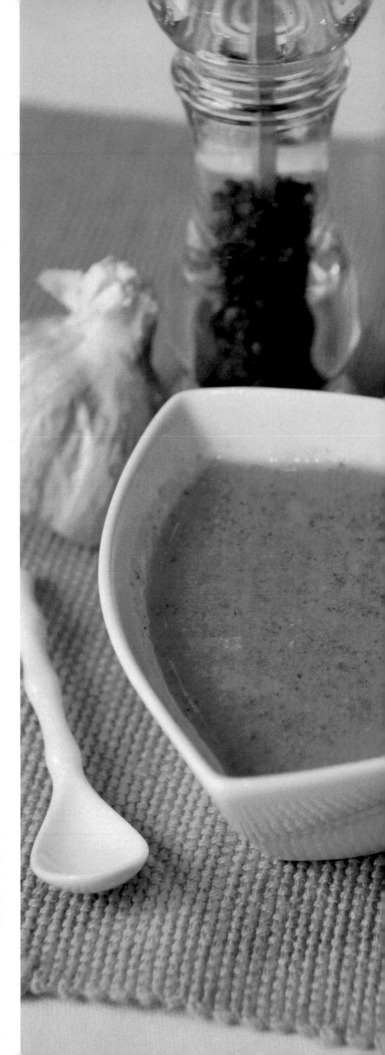

Smooth Pureed Diet

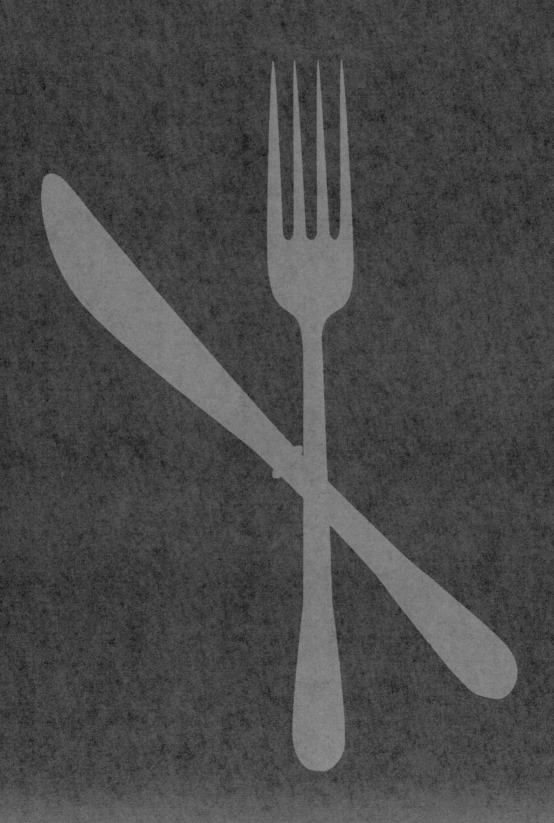

Recovery Stage 2: Smooth Pureed Diet

Following the fluid diet, thicker foods can start to be included. Smooth pureed foods should be smooth and moist with no lumps, like the texture of smooth mashed potato.

On the smooth pureed diet, suitable foods are the texture of a smooth, mashed potato.

Many foods can be pureed in a food processor or blender to form this texture. Some foods are a suitable texture without pureeing, for example low fat yoghurt, custard or baby food. Baby food is convenient, but contains inadequate nutrition for an adult. It is therefore not a substitute for homemade food.

Remain on the smooth pureed diet for as long as your surgical team recommends.

The different types of surgery have different effects on the stomach. Depending on the surgery you have had, your surgeon's technique and your individual recovery, you will be given specific recommendations for the time required to stay on a smooth pureed diet after surgery.

A *Smooth Pureed Diet Sample Menu* is provided (page 77) and our surgical team suggest you follow this for two weeks. This is a suggestion only. If your support team recommends differently, follow their advice.

As the food you are eating becomes thicker you will need to allow more time to eat. Eat slowly, allowing up to 20 minutes to eat a small meal. Take note of when you start to feel satisfied and stop eating. Always stop eating if you feel any discomfort.

Protein on the smooth pureed diet

Protein is used to build and repair the body and your body will continue to heal during the smooth pureed diet. Some protein-containing foods may be difficult to puree, as they are too dry and stringy, such as grilled meat and chicken. When pureeing meat, extra fluid is needed. Foods that are easiest to puree are moist, such as casseroles, stews or mornays. These can be pureed, split into smaller portions and frozen, ready to heat and eat.

The *Smooth Pureed Foods* recipes (from page 78) includes a range of recipe suggestions that are good sources of protein.

Best Choices: Smooth Pureed Foods High in Protein
(choose for meals)

- *Smooth Pureed Foods* (from page 78)
- pureed casseroles, stews or mornays containing meat, chicken, fish or legumes
- pureed baked beans
- lightly scrambled eggs* (not hard or lumpy)
- low fat yoghurt, in particular, Chobani® yoghurt
- low fat custard
- smooth, low fat cottage cheese
- smooth, low fat ricotta cheese

Include Less Often: Smooth Pureed Foods Low in Protein
(include with a food high in protein)

- smooth, mashed vegetables eg. potato, sweet potato, pumpkin
- pureed fruits

Some people will not tolerate scrambled eggs in the first few weeks following surgery, particularly those who have had a sleeve gastrectomy. Discuss with your dietitian.

Everyone will have a different recovery after surgery. You may not be able to eat all the foods recommended on the smooth pureed diet menu as everyone has a different capacity. After sleeve gastrectomy and gastric bypass surgeries, you will tolerate smaller amounts than those who have had gastric band surgery. To make sure you are getting adequate protein to help you recover, include a VLED or BODIE'z product each day and the higher protein purees from the menu. See the nutrition information provided with each recipe to choose the higher protein options. You can also use whey protein isolate powders to add additional protein to your fluids and purees. Speak to your dietitian about how much protein powder would be appropriate to meet your individual needs each day.

Some smoothies from the fluid diet can be included on the puree diet for variety. However, as you progress through the textures, you should choose the thicker, or more solid options where you can as these will be more satisfying.

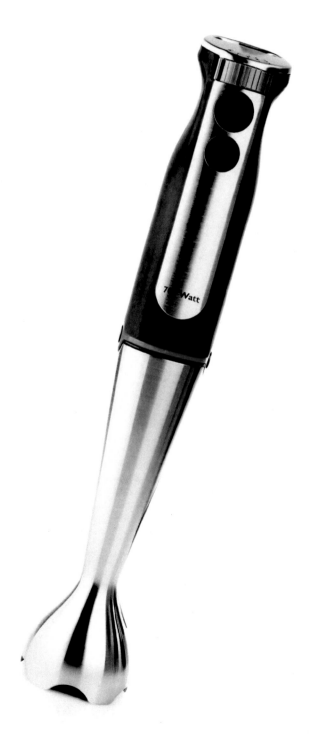

SMOOTH PUREE DIET SAMPLE MENU

Breakfast Options

- Weetbix® made with warm milk and mashed until smooth
- Scrambled Egg (page 79)
- Apple & Apricot (page 80)
- Pear & Ricotta Whip (page 87)
- Mango & Yoghurt (page 88)
- Chobani® yoghurt

Lunch Options

- Scrambled Egg (page 79)
- Creamy Chicken Casserole (page 209)
- Salmon & Avocado Mousse (page 82)
- Tomato, Lentils & Vegetables (page 83)
- Creamy Mixed Vegetables with Nutmeg (page 84)
- Fish & Sweet Potato (page 85)
- Italian Style Chicken (page 86)
- Shepherd's Pie (page 89)

Dinner Options

As for Lunch Options

Mid Morning, Mid Afternoon and Supper

As per the Fluid Diet Menu, sip on any of the suggested smoothies, milk based coffee, VLED milkshakes or BODIE'z clear protein water* as tolerated.

BODIE'z clear protein waters are available at www.bodiezpro.com. When placing an order be sure to use our Nutrition for Weight Loss Surgery discount code, NFWLS.

Using the Smooth Pureed Recipes

Serving sizes

The smooth pureed recipes are designed to make approximately two, one cup serves.

Immediately following sleeve gastrectomy and gastric bypass surgery, you may only tolerate one quarter of a cup at a time.

Immediately following gastric band surgery, you may only tolerate half a cup at one time. As your swelling subsides, some may tolerate one cup.

Everyone recovers differently and will tolerate different amounts. If you only tolerate small amounts, make sure you include a VLED product or BODIE'z protein water each day and choose the higher protein puree recipes. See the nutrition information provided with each recipe to choose the higher protein options. You can also use additional whey protein isolate powders to add additional protein to your fluids and purees.

Regardless of the surgery you have had, eat slowly and stop before you feel any discomfort.

Most of the smooth pureed recipes are suitable to freeze. Use small freezer bags or containers to freeze in single serves if you only tolerate small amounts.

Whilst the thought of smooth pureed recipes may not appeal to family and friends, some can be used as appealing accompaniments to other dishes. For example, Creamy Mixed Vegetables with Nutmeg (page 84) makes a tasty accompaniment to a grilled steak with some steamed green vegetables such as zucchini, broccoli or snow peas.

Hints and tips

Throughout the recipes, practical hints and tips are included between the yellow lines.

> "I found the whole book very useful but if you'd like me to narrow it down to specific sections I liked the Smooth Pureed Foods. "
>
> *- Sandra, gastric band -*

Scrambled Egg

Makes 2 cups

Oil spray

2 eggs

4 tablespoons low fat milk or low fat evaporated milk

Heat a small saucepan that has been sprayed with oil. Beat egg and add milk. Add to the saucepan and heat gently, moving mixture gently so it can cook through. Do not allow to boil or brown. Cook until set. Alternatively, the mixture can be cooked in a small, microwave-proof bowl. Cook on medium to high heat for 60-90 seconds, stirring every 30 seconds. Take care not to overcook eggs as they need to remain soft, without lumps, whilst on the smooth pureed diet.

Nutrition information (per cup): kilojoules 865, calories 207, protein 16.5g, fat 13.5g, saturated fat 3.5g, carbohydrate 5.5g, fibre nil.

Serve scrambled eggs on wholegrain/multigrain toast for family and friends. Add an extra 2 eggs and 4 tablespoons of milk per person.

> "This is easy to do, particularly for a lunch meal. At the beginning of the Smooth Puree Diet, I found one egg to be quite filling."
> - Lisi, gastric bypass -

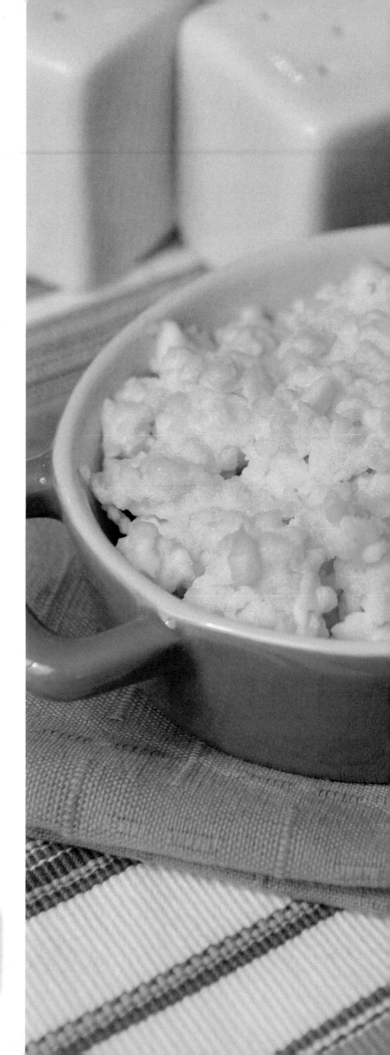

Apple & Apricot

Makes 2 cups

2 apples, peeled, cored and chopped

6 dried apricots, chopped

100g soft tofu

2 tablespoons almond meal

1 tablespoon (15g) whey protein isolate powder

Pinch of cinnamon (optional)

Place apples and apricots in a pan and cover with water. Bring to the boil, reduce heat, cover and simmer for about 5-10 minutes or until apples and apricots are soft. Drain apricot and apple and reserve liquid. Combine apricot, apple, tofu and almond meal in a blender and puree until smooth. Add enough reserved cooking liquid whilst pureeing to make the texture of the mixture like smooth, mashed potato. Add protein powder and blend on low speed until combined. Add cinnamon to taste.

Nutrition information (per cup): kilojoules 1030, calories 246, protein 15.5g, fat 8.5g, saturated fat 1g, carbohydrate 25.5g, fibre 5.5g.

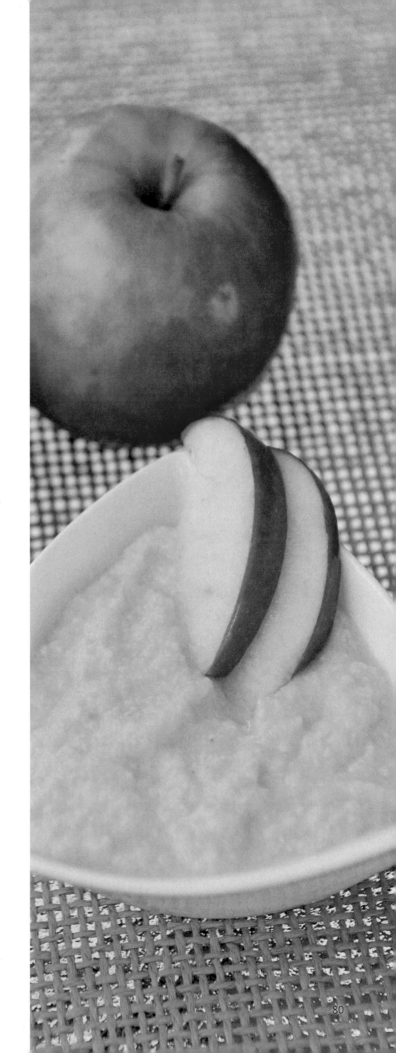

Creamy Chicken & Vegetables

Makes 2 cups

Oil spray

1 clove garlic, crushed

1 onion, diced

200g skinless chicken, trimmed of fat, diced

1 celery stick, finely diced

1 carrot, peeled and diced

½ cup cauliflower, diced

½ cup sweet potato, peeled and diced

2 cups salt reduced chicken stock

¼ cup Philadelphia® extra light cream cheese

Pinch of tarragon (optional)

Heat a saucepan that has been sprayed with oil. Add onion, garlic and chicken and cook for 3-4 minutes. Add the vegetables and pour over the stock. Bring to the boil and simmer, covered for about 30 minutes or until the chicken is cooked through and the vegetables are tender. Drain and reserve liquid. Pour mixture into a blender or food processor and add cream cheese. Sprinkle with tarragon if desired. Puree until smooth, adding enough cooking liquid to make the texture of the mixture like smooth, mashed potato.

Nutrition Information: kilojoules 1280, calories 306, protein 30g, fat 11.5g, saturated fat 4g, carbohydrate 17.5g, fibre 3.5g.

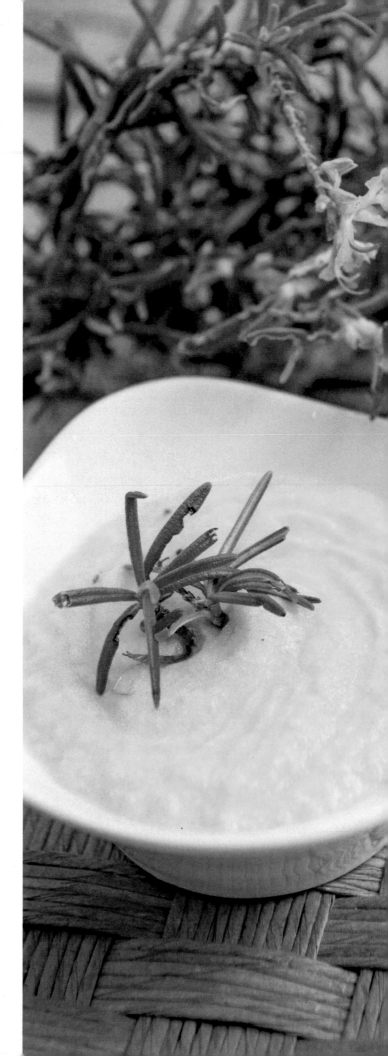

Salmon & Avocado Mousse

Serves 4

Avocado layer

1 ripe avocado

2 level teaspoons gelatine, dissolved in ¼ cup hot water

2 tablespoons lemon juice

½ teaspoon dried dill

Couple of drops of Tabasco

Salmon layer

2 x 130g tins of premium skinless, boneless salmon

2 level teaspoons of gelatine, dissolved in ¼ cup hot water

¼ cup low fat mayonnaise

Couple of drops of Tabasco

To make the avocado layer, mash the avocado until smooth. Add lemon juice, dill and Tabasco and mix well. Dissolve the gelatine and add to the avocado mix. Layer the avocado mixture in small glasses or bowls and refrigerate. To make the salmon layer, blend the tinned salmon, including the liquid, with a blender or food processor. Add the mayonnaise and Tabasco and combine well. Dissolve the gelatine in the hot water and stir through the salmon mixture. Layer on top of avocado, cover with glad wrap and refrigerate over night.

Nutrition information (per serve): kilojoules 1020, calories 358, protein 15.5g, fat 17.5g, saturated fat 4g, carbohydrate 5.5g, fibre 2g.

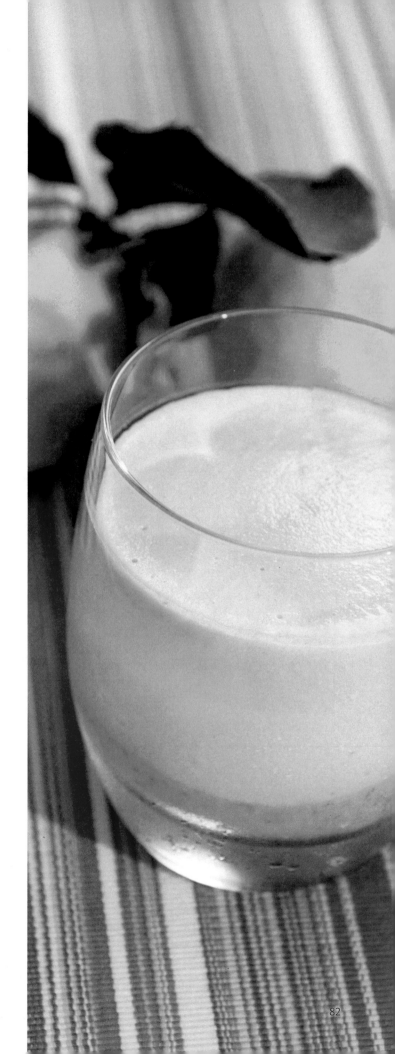

Tomato Lentils & Vegetables

Makes 2 cups

Oil spray

1 clove garlic, crushed

½ onion, finely diced

½ small zucchini, diced

½ stick celery, finely diced

½ cup eggplant, diced

¼ cup dry red lentils, washed

½ cup sweet potato, peeled and diced

1 cup salt reduced vegetable stock

½ cup no added salt tomato puree

2 tablespoons (30g) whey protein isolate powder

Pinch of parsley and/or basil

Heat a small saucepan that has been sprayed with oil. Add onion and garlic and cook until soft. Add lentils and stock. Bring to the boil. Reduce heat and simmer, covered, for 10 minutes. Add zucchini, sweet potato, celery, eggplant and tomato puree. Simmer until the vegetables are soft. Drain mixture and reserve liquid. Place mixture in a blender and sprinkle with parsley and/or basil. Puree mixture until smooth, adding cooking liquid as necessary to make the texture of the mixture like smooth, mashed potato. Use a little of the remaining cooking liquid to dissolve the whey protein isolate powder. Stir the dissolved powder through the pureed mixture until combined.

Nutrition information (per cup): kilojoules 890, calories 213, protein 22g, fat 3.5g, saturated fat 0.5g, carbohydrate 20.5g, fibre 6.5g.

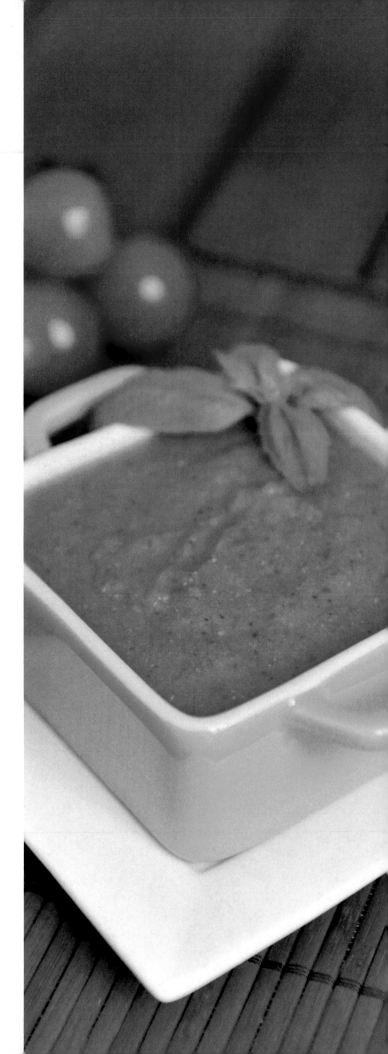

Creamy Mixed Vegetables with Nutmeg

Makes 2 cups

1 cup carrot, peeled and diced

½ cup swede, peeled and diced

1 cup pumpkin, peeled and diced

½ cup parsnip, peeled and diced

3 tablespoons dry red lentils, washed

1½ cups low fat milk

Pinch of nutmeg

Freshly ground black pepper

Add vegetables, lentils and milk to a saucepan. Bring to a gentle simmer, and cook for approximately 20 minutes or until the vegetables are tender. Stir regularly to prevent milk forming a skin. Drain mixture and reserve liquid. Place mixture in a blender or food processor and sprinkle with nutmeg. Puree mixture until smooth, adding cooking liquid as necessary to make the texture of the mixture like smooth, mashed potato. Season to taste with freshly ground black pepper.

Nutrition information (per cup): kilojoules 945, calories 226, protein 17.5g, fat 1g, saturated fat 0.5g, carbohydrate 33.5g, fibre 8g.

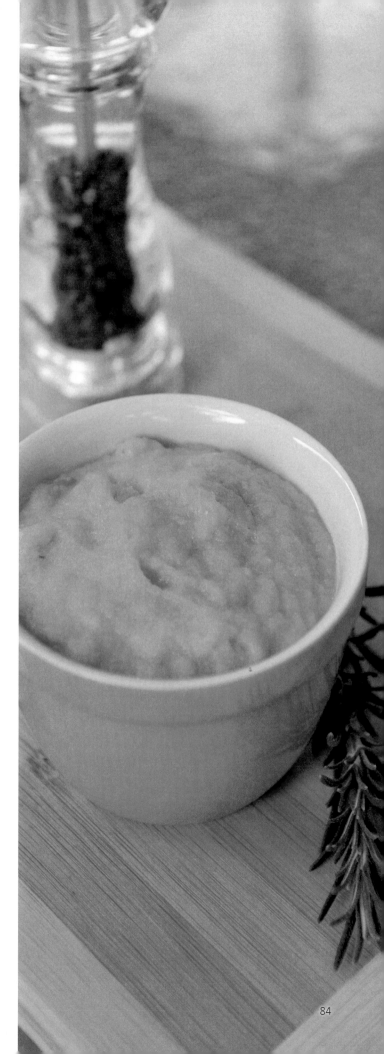

Fish & Sweet Potato

Makes 2 cups

2 cups sweet potato, peeled and diced

200g white fish

¼ cup lemon juice

Place sweet potato into a saucepan and cover with water. Bring to the boil then cover and simmer for 10-15 minutes or until just soft. Add fish and cook 5 minutes, or until the fish is cooked through. Drain mixture. Pour fish and sweet potato into a blender or food processor. Puree mixture until smooth, adding 1-2 tablespoons of lemon juice as necessary to make the texture of the mixture like smooth, mashed potato.

Nutrition information (per cup): kilojoules 875, calories 209, protein 23.5g, fat 2.5g, saturated fat 0.5g, carbohydrate 21g, fibre 2.5g.

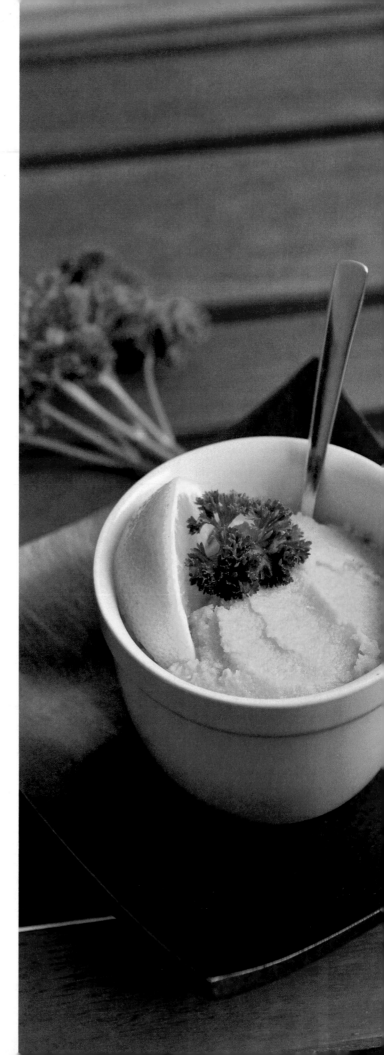

Italian Style Chicken

Makes 2 cups

Oil spray

1 clove garlic, crushed

½ onion, chopped

1 zucchini, diced (approx 1 cup)

200g chicken, trimmed of fat, diced
eg. breast, thigh or tenderloin

1/2 cup eggplant, diced

2 heaped tablespoons roasted capsicum, diced

1 mushroom, diced

¾ cup no added salt, chopped tinned tomatoes

½ cup salt reduced chicken stock

Pinch of basil and oregano

Heat a saucepan that has been sprayed with oil. Add onion and garlic and cook until soften. Add chicken and cook until seared on all sides. Add zucchini, eggplant, capsicum and mushroom and cook for a few minutes. Add the chopped tomatoes and stock. Bring to the boil and cook over low heat for approximately 20 minutes or until the potato is quite soft. Drain the chicken and vegetables and reserve the liquid. Add basil and oregano. Add to a blender and puree until smooth. Add enough reserved cooking liquid whilst pureeing to make the texture of the mixture like smooth, mashed potato.

Nutrition information (per cup): kilojoules 860, calories 205, protein 21g, fat 11g, saturated fat 3g, carbohydrate 7g, fibre 2.5g.

"This was beautiful!"
- Simon, gastric band -

"This puree was full of flavour and the addition of stock made it easy to control the texture."
- Robyn, gastric bypass -

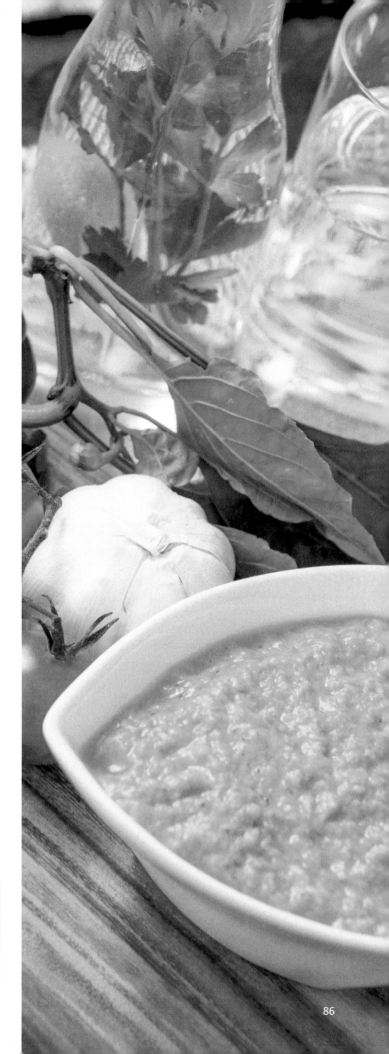

Pear & Ricotta Whip

Makes 2 cups

1 cup canned pear in natural juice, diced and drained, juice reserved

1 cup reduced fat firm ricotta cheese

1 tablespoon (15g) whey protein isolate powder

Sprinkle of cinnamon

Add pear to a blender or food processor and puree. Whilst pureeing, add reserved pear juice, 1 tablespoon at a time, to ensure the texture is smooth. Set aside in a glass. Add ricotta and protein powder to a blender or food processor and puree. Whilst pureeing, add reserved pear juice, 1 tablespoon at a time, to ensure the texture is smooth. Layer on top of pear. Sprinkle with cinnamon if desired.

Nutrition information (per cup): kilojoules 1080, calories 258, protein 21g, fat 11.5g, saturated fat 7.5g, carbohydrate 18g, fibre 2g.

Pear and Ricotta Whip makes an excellent whipped cream substitute. Simply puree all the ingredients together. Serve this whip with strawberries or sliced fresh fruit as a dessert for family and friends.

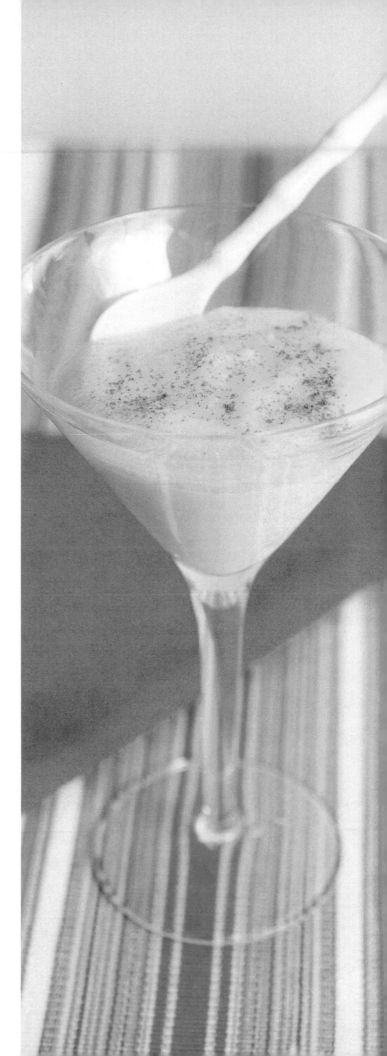

Mango & Yoghurt

Makes 2 cups

1 cup canned mango in natural juice, drained

1 cup Chobani® plain low fat yoghurt

2 tablespoons almond meal

Place mango in a blender or food processor and puree until smooth. Combine almond meal and yoghurt and mix well. Fold pureed mango gently through yoghurt.

Nutrition information (per cup): kilojoules 855, calories 205, protein 15.5g, fat 7g, saturated fat 1.5g, carbohydrate 18.5g, fibre 2g.

- Mango can be replaced with other soft fruit. Tinned fruit in natural juice will puree easily. Experiment with canned pears, peaches or apple for variety.

- Chobani® plain low fat yoghurt is used in this recipe as it is a readily available, higher protein yoghurt. You can use other brands of plain or vanilla yoghurt in this recipe, however it is likely they will be lower in protein and often higher in sugar.

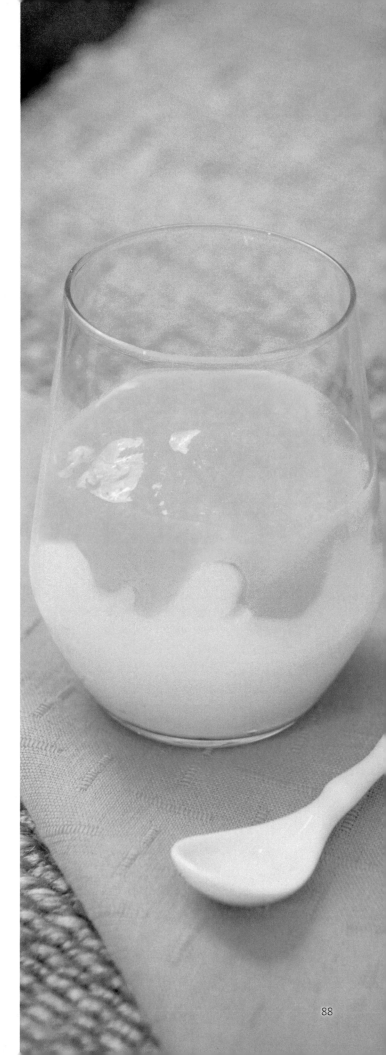

Shepherd's Pie

Makes 2 cups

Oil spray

1 clove garlic, crushed

1 onion, diced

200g lean lamb or beef mince

1 stick celery, finely diced

1 carrot, diced

1 cup salt reduced beef stock

1 tablespoon no added salt tomato paste

2 teaspoons Worcestershire sauce

½ cup potato, diced

½ cup sweet potato, diced

1-2 tablespoons milk

Preheat oven to 200°C. Heat a saucepan that has been sprayed with oil. Add onion, garlic and mince and brown. Add remaining ingredients, except potatoes and milk, to the saucepan and bring to the boil. Cover and simmer until vegetables are soft and the liquid has reduced slightly. Drain and reserve liquid. Add the meat and vegetable mixture to a blender and puree. Add enough reserved cooking liquid while pureeing to ensure the texture of the mixture like smooth, mashed potato. Cook potatoes in a saucepan of boiling water for 15 minutes or until they are tender. Drain well. Use a potato masher or fork to mash. Add milk and use a wooden spoon to stir until combined into a smooth texture. Add meat mixture to a small ramekin or oven proof dish and layer potato mixture on top. Spray with oil spray. Bake in the oven for 15 minutes or until golden on top.

Nutrition information (per cup): kilojoules 1500, calories 358, protein 31.5g, fat 14g, saturated fat 5.5g, carbohydrate 23g, fibre 4.5g.

"This is a good recipe to get the meat taste in the diet. This is very easy for taking to work to heat up for lunch."

- Lisi, gastric bypass -

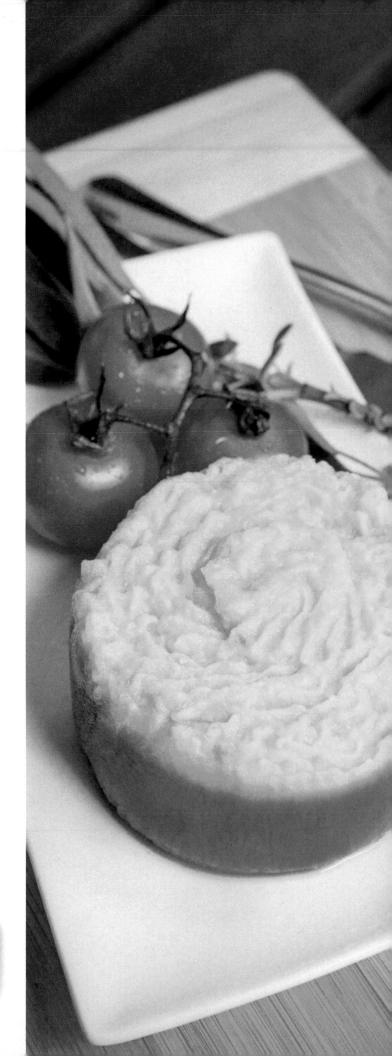

Soft Diet

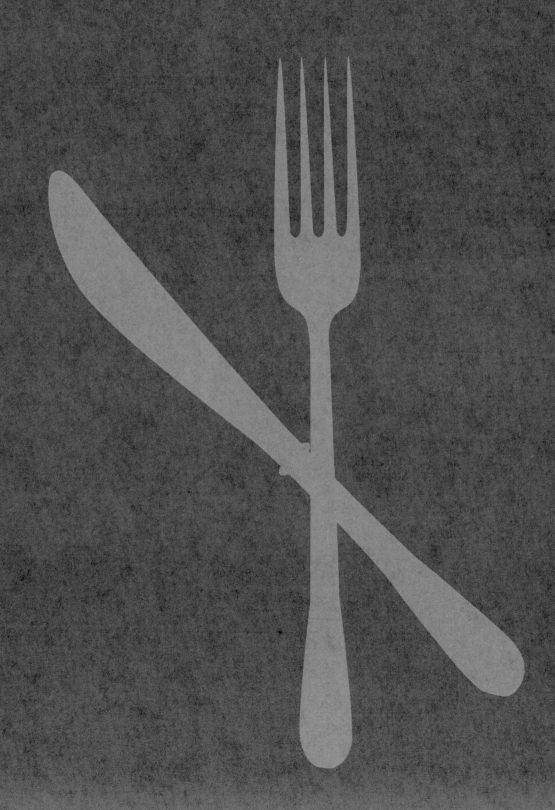

Recovery Stage 3: Soft Diet

Following the fluid and smooth pureed diets, much of your swelling will have subsided. The soft diet allows you to experiment with some 'normal' foods as you progress back to a diet of solid food.

Soft foods can be mashed with a fork and can be chewed until they feel like a puree in the mouth before swallowing. For example, grilled fish or shepherd's pie can be cut with a fork and chewed to a smooth puree, but a well-done steak cannot.

On the soft diet, suitable foods can be broken with the side of a fork, or chewed into a puree in the mouth before swallowing.

Some foods are not easy to chew into a smooth puree in the mouth and you should delay trying these. These include:

- tough or chewy meat, such as barbequed or grilled meat or chicken breast
- stringy foods, such as celery or fresh asparagus
- doughy foods, such as fresh white bread
- tough skins, seeds and pith on fruit and vegetables
- raw vegetables and salad such as carrot, lettuce, cabbage and corn.

Following a sleeve gastrectomy or gastric bypass you are also best to avoid rice and pasta at this stage, as it can swell up in the new stomach and make you feel bloated and uncomfortable. They can also take the place of protein-containing foods that are important in your recovery.

Remain on the soft diet for as long as your surgical team recommends.

The different types of surgery have different effects on the stomach. Depending on the surgery you have and your surgeon's technique, he or she will have specific recommendations for the time required to stay on a soft diet after surgery.

The soft diet is a transition phase and some 'normal' foods can be included, hence separate recipes for the soft diet are not provided. However, a sample menu of recipes suitable for the soft diet from the *Recipes for Healthy Living* section is provided on page 118.

The recipes suitable for a soft diet are indicated with the **S** icon throughout the *Recipes for Healthy Living section*.

Protein on the soft diet

Those who have had sleeve gastrectomy or gastric bypass surgery will eat smaller amounts following surgery than those with a gastric band. Speak to your dietitian to make sure you are getting adequate protein to help you recover. When you eat your meals, make sure you eat the protein-containing part of the meal first.

As you are able to include more solid protein-containing foods you can reduce your intake of VLED milkshakes, soups and smoothies. Solid foods are best long term to help you feel satisfied after eating which will help to achieve your weight loss goals.

Tips for a soft diet

The following tips will help you experiment with foods from all food groups on the soft diet.

TIPS FOR A SOFT DIET AND REINTRODUCING 'NORMAL' FOODS

Meat and meat alternatives

- Start with fish, eggs and lean minced meats on a soft diet.
- Slow cook meat or chicken in stews or casseroles to tenderise them. Slow cookers work well, however, you can achieve similar results by cooking casseroles on the stove or in the oven on low heat for several hours
- Once you are comfortable with stews and casseroles, try roasted meats, sliced thinly, with gravy or sauce. Allow the gravy or sauce to soak into the meat fibres to help soften them before eating.
- Always cut meat or chicken across the grain.
- Either marinate, or serve meat and chicken with gravy or sauce.
- Tofu and legumes can also be included as softer meat alternatives, however they are much lower in protein than meats, so make it more challenging to meet your protein requirements. Discuss with your dietitian.

Milk and milk products

- Cheeses can be included in a soft diet.
- Continue to include reduced or low fat milk and yoghurts, however you can rely on them less than during the fluid and smooth pureed stages as a range of foods from different food groups can now be introduced.

Breads, cereals, rice, pasta and noodles*

- Avoid fresh bread initially. Try wholemeal or grainy cracker biscuits, flat bread such as mountain bread or thin wraps and toast before trying fresh bread. These are generally less doughy and easier to chew to a puree in the mouth.
- Allow cereals to soak a little in milk. Choose the high fibre varieties such as porridge, Weetbix®, etc.
- Make sure rice is moist. Try dishes such as risotto, or serve rice with a moist sauce or topping such as a casserole or curry. Delay trying dry rice such as sushi or fried rice until later.
- Dry or 'sticky' pasta should be avoided. Serve well-cooked pasta with a moist sauce and mix well. Choose tomato-based sauces but don't forget the protein. Include lean mince, chicken, tuna or legumes.

In the early stages following sleeve gastrectomy and gastric bypass, bread, pasta and rice can swell in the new, smaller stomach and cause pain and discomfort. These foods can interfere with the intake of protein-containing foods, which are important to help your recovery. If you have diabetes, it is important to include some carbohydrate-containing foods. However, legumes, milk and milk products may be more comfortable to eat and will also provide you with protein. If you are unsure about your intake of these foods or your individual carbohydrate needs, speak with your dietitian.

TIPS FOR A SOFT DIET AND REINTRODUCING 'NORMAL' FOODS

Vegetables*

- Cook vegetables until they are soft enough to be cut with the side of a fork. As you feel ready, try them crisper.
- If oven baking vegetables, remove tough skins such as those on pumpkin or potato.
- Slice stringy vegetables such as celery or asparagus very finely to break the strings, and then use them in casseroles or stews.
- When you feel ready, cut or 'shred' salad vegetables finely on the plate before eating. Even though lettuce is not 'tough', the small fibres should be broken up so they don't hold together.
- Try using some canned vegetables as part of your salads as these are often a little softer. For example, tinned corn makes a tasty and colourful addition to salads and is easy to chew.
- Try cooking vegetables to add to salads. Roast strips of capsicum, eggplant or zucchini to to make them more tender then add to your salads.

*In the early stages following sleeve gastrectomy or gastric bypass, be careful not to fill up on these foods. Always eat protein-containing foods first.

Fruit

- Try soft, ripe fruits such as ripe banana or pear, rockmelon or mango.
- Peel tough skins on fruit such as kiwi fruit and peaches.
- Tinned fruits in natural juice are soft and easy to chew.
- When you feel ready, slice harder fruits such as apples into thin slices before eating.

SOFT DIET SAMPLE MENU

Breakfast Options

- Weetbix® soaked with milk until soft
- Bircher Muesli (page 126)
- Bacon & Egg Breakfast Muffins (page 127)
- Mushroom, Rocket & Tomato Omelette (page 135)
- Nutty Chia Porridge (page 130)
- Baked beans
- Chobani® yoghurt and soft fruit.

Lunch Options

- Pumpkin & Spinach Frittata (page 139)
- Chunky Winter Soup (page 140)
- Baked beans
- Tuna & Sweet Potato Frittatas (page 147)
- Zucchini Slice (page 149)
- Scrambled egg.

Dinner Options

- Zesty Tomato Fish (page 171)
- Meatballs with Vegetable Sauce (page 181)
- Creamy Vegetable Curry (page 187)
- Chicken Creole (page 191)
- Tasty Tomato Beef (page 189)
- Pumpkin, Spinach & Ricotta Cannelloni (page 195)
- Baked Salmon with Cauliflower Puree (page 177)
- Slow Cooked Lamb Curry (page 207)
- Chicken Curry (page 197)
- Bean & Vegetable Hot Pot (page 178)
- Middle Eastern Lamb (page 185).

Mid Morning, Mid Afternoon and Supper

As your meals become more solid, you may no longer need to have the smaller, between meal snacks. Start to tune in to your hunger and satiety signals. You may find a drink containing protein is enough, for example milk based coffee or BODIE'z protein water. If you do feel you need a snack, consider the softer options of the snack ideas listed on page on page 107.

Important Points for all Stages of Recovery

Fluid

It is important to keep hydrated during your recovery. Low energy fluids such as water, tea or diet cordial should be sipped between meals to keep you hydrated. Try to include at least 1500mL (1½L) of fluid in small, regular amounts spread throughout the day. All fluids can contribute to this total. Drink slowly and stop before you feel any discomfort.

Avoid fizzy drinks. The gas in fizzy drinks may be uncomfortable following surgery. Some people experience these symptoms long term so should avoid fizzy drinks permanently.

For those who have had a sleeve gastrectomy or gastric bypass, your new, smaller stomach will not fit food and fluid at the same time. Leave 30 minutes between eating and drinking.

Remind yourself to drink often; carry a water bottle with you, keep a jug of water on your desk at work or in a place where you walk past it often at home. If you find plain water difficult, add diet cordial or try herbal tea. To help meet both your fluid and protein requirements, consider BODIE'z clear protein waters. These are available online at www.bodiezpro.com. Be sure to use our discount code, NFWLS, when you place an order.

Vitamin and mineral supplements

Whilst the aim of surgery is to take in less energy (calories or kilojoules) and therefore lose weight, your body still requires adequate vitamins and minerals. Remember to include the vitamins and mineral supplements recommended by your team. For more information on vitamin and mineral supplements see the *Nutritional Impacts of Weight Loss Surgery and Supplementation* chapter (page 232).

Fibre

The amount of food you are now eating is much less than before surgery, so it is likely you will use your bowels less. As long as you are not uncomfortable, this is not a problem.

During the fluid diet and smooth pureed diets it can be difficult to obtain enough fibre and constipation can occur.

When on the fluid diet, soups with lots of vegetables that have been pureed until they are smooth will increase your fibre intake; however, remember that fluids must be thin enough to pass through a straw. On the smooth pureed diet, fibrous foods must also be pureed until they are smooth, like the texture of smooth, mashed potato. On the soft diet you can get fibre from soft fruits, vegetables and cereals. Soft fruits such as ripe banana, pear and peach are good examples of an appropriate texture for fruit during the soft diet stage. Well-cooked vegetables and wholegrain cereals moistened with milk also help to increase fibre intake. Longer-term, including wholemeal or wholegrain/multigrain products and cereals, fruit, vegetables, and ensuring adequate fluids and regular exercise will assist with regular bowel motions.

If you are constipated at any stage, you may find a fibre supplement useful. A soluble fibre supplement such as Benefiber® may be useful as it is colourless and tasteless, hence can be dissolved in a range of fluids. A small glass of prune or pear juice daily may also help.

Dehydration also causes constipation so try to include at least 1500mL (1½L) of fluid daily. If constipation persists, discuss this with your surgical team or GP. Please seek medical advice before commencing laxatives.

Living with
Weight Loss Surgery

Food Fundamentals Following Weight Loss Surgery

Living with Weight Loss Surgery

Are we there yet?

No! It is now that the real journey begins. First the VLED program, followed by the fluid and smooth pureed diets are necessary for a safe surgery and recovery, it is now up to you to put in place the healthy lifestyle to achieve your goals. The journey to better health involves losing a significant amount of weight. This is not always easy on your own.

Studies show that those who regularly attend more follow-up appointments with their team, including the dietitian, lose more weight. Follow up with your whole team is important, not just your surgeon.

What can a Dietitian do?

Dietitians don't just help people lose weight. Some people who have weight loss surgery will have medical conditions with specific dietary needs. In Australia, only an Accredited Practising Dietitian (APD) is qualified to advise on the nutritional management of chronic health conditions such as diabetes, heart disease, gastrointestinal disorders and food allergy and intolerance.

APDs will often distinguish themselves with the words Accredited Practising Dietitian or the following logo:

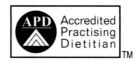

APDs can educate patients, families, partners and carers on life after weight loss surgery to achieve weight loss. They can also help with advice on:

- obtaining all the nutrients needed for good health
- managing specific health conditions
- vitamin and mineral supplementation
- eating more comfortably
- getting enough protein
- preventing nutrient deficiencies
- managing hunger
- mindful eating
- dining out and takeaway foods
- snacks
- practical meal ideas
- meal planning and shopping
- reading and understanding food labels
- recipe modification.

Long-term success following weight loss surgery involves changes to many aspects of your life. If your surgical team does not include an APD, ask for a referral to one. Alternatively you can find an Accredited Practising Dietitian who is experienced in weight loss surgery using the *Find a Dietitian* link on the Obesity Surgery Society of Australia and New Zealand website (www.ossanz.com.au).

> "To help stay motivated, keep going to your appointments with the dietitian, doctor and psychologist... You may think you don't need to (like I did) but they really do help!"
>
> - Elise, gastric band -

Prepare, serve and eat small amounts of food

Weight loss surgery helps you to feel satisfied on a smaller amount of food. You will therefore need to prepare and serve small amounts of food.

Surgeons will differ in their recommendations of how much food you should be eating. Some may say limit meals to half a cup, some may say one cup, and others will say a bread and butter plate of food. Interestingly, one cup of food nicely fits on a bread and butter plate and this is the guide we use in our clinic.

Accredited Practising Dietitians are university-qualified experts on food and nutrition. What they will generally agree on is that it is difficult to meet your nutritional requirements in half a cup of food, three times a day. For this reason it is vital that you include vitamin and mineral supplements as recommended by your team, or as described in the *Nutritional Impacts of Weight Loss Surgery and Supplementation* chapter (page 232).

To date, there are no scientific studies on the exact amount of food people should include after gastric band and gastric bypass surgeries. Hopefully in time this will evolve. Your surgical team has seen many people who undergo these surgeries and hence have an understanding of the amount of food most people will tolerate comfortably. Be guided by your team and always stop eating before you feel any discomfort.

Research from Mercy Bariatrics in Perth, Western Australia, provides some excellent data to help guide serving sizes for those who have had a sleeve gastrectomy. Over time your sleeve will get used to a little more food. At six months after surgery, you will manage about half a cup of food at a time. By 12 to 18 months you will manage about one cup of solid food. This is a guide only and will vary between people. The people studied found they could indeed 'fit' more food in than what they felt satisfied with, however, eating to the maximum amount you can tolerate is not recommended. Over time this can stretch the sleeve, defeating the purpose of the surgery. It is important to note that surgeons will create sleeves of different sizes and individual experiences will vary.

Whilst there is little hard evidence in this area, what you will generally find is that those who have a sleeve gastrectomy or gastric bypass will start by eating very small amounts in the early stages following surgery and over time this will increase. Whereas once the initial swelling subsides after gastric band surgery, some people find they can eat larger amounts and it takes some time before they feel satisfied on small amounts of food. Many people need their gastric band adjusted several times to help them feel satisfied on small serves. If small meals of solid food do not satisfy you, keep in regular contact with your support team until they do. Some people will find this will occur early in their journey, for others it may take longer. Be patient.

Throughout this book, most of the recipes have been designed to provide approximately four, one cup serves (except the Low Energy Vegetables and Smooth Pureed Foods). This does not mean that we think you should always eat one cup of food. It just means that once you learn how much food is generally comfortable for you to eat at a meal, you to easily adapt the recipes to your requirements.

As was mentioned earlier regarding the study on the capacity of sleeves, people could 'fit' more food than what they felt satisfied eating. This is such an important point to emphasise as it is relevant to all forms of surgery. People who have had surgery often compare stories on how much food they can fit in. It is important to understand that eating is not a competition and seeing how much you can fit at any one time should not be your goal. Testing your limits and overeating can cause complications after all forms of surgery and most certainly does not help weight loss or weight maintenance long term. Below is one of my favourite quotes from bariatric GP Teresa Girolamo:

> "It's not about seeing how much you can eat and get away, but how little you can eat and feel satisfied."

This should be your goal. Tune in to the signals from your body to understand how much food you can enjoy comfortably whilst managing your hunger.

The following tips can be useful to help you eat small amounts of food:

- Create an environment that makes it easy for you to eat small portions. Ensure family and friends know you use a smaller plate, bowl and cutlery. Take these items with you if you travel.
- Cook food and freeze in small portions. Use small containers, zip lock bags or muffin trays to freeze foods in an appropriate size for you.
- When eating out, order entrée size meals or if there are none available, separate your meal into an appropriate portion before you start eating. Tapas style menus, Asian or Indian eateries are often tailored to meals being shared, allowing you to dish up a small serve to suit your needs.
- It is fine to leave food on your plate when you have had enough, even if it is a smaller serve.
- Avoid the temptation to 'clean the plate'. In most cases, 'cleaning the plate' is deliberately overriding your internal signals.
- Serve less food rather than more. If you are still hungry you can always eat something else, but stop and think before you do, rather than eating it automatically without thinking.

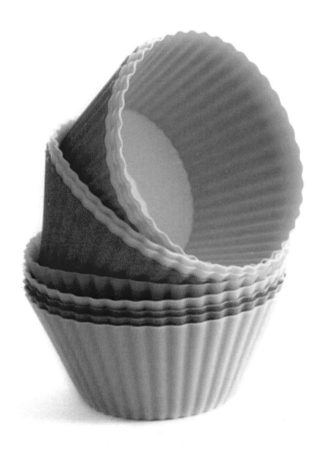

Eat slowly and mindfully

We used to always talk to our weight loss surgery clients about eating slowly, but in recent times we have expanded this to include eating mindfully. Mindful eating has gained traction as an important concept in healthy eating and weight management. Eating slowly allows you to eat mindfully, so it is only natural that we focus on these concepts together.

In the short term, eating too quickly after weight loss surgery means that you are unlikely to chew foods properly, which may cause discomfort and/ or pain. Longer term however, it means you are unlikely to gain an awareness of the signals your body is giving you regarding your hunger and satiety and understanding these signals are key factors in long term weight management.

If you focus firstly on slowing down your eating, you can then start to incorporate mindful eating. After weight loss surgery, it should take around 10 minutes to eat a small meal. For some it may take a little longer. If you have trouble slowing down your eating, put your cutlery down between mouthfuls. Wait until you have swallowed your food before cutting the next piece. Avoid having that next mouthful loaded on your fork ready to go. If you really struggle to slow down, use your cutlery in the opposite hand until the pace of eating feels more natural.

Whilst eating slowly is important, so is knowing when to stop. If there is food left on your plate after 20 minutes, discard it. Spending too long eating meals can mean meals turn into long grazing episodes, which should also be avoided.

One of the experts in the mindful eating field, Michelle May, defines mindful eating as "eating with intention and attention".

To eat with intention is about being purposeful when you eat, for example:

- Eating when you are truly hungry.
- Eating to meet your body's needs by choosing foods that are nourishing and satisfying.
- Eating with the goal of feeling better when you're finished than you did when you started.

To eat with attention means devoting your full attention to eating, including

- Eliminating or minimising distractions.
- Tuning into the flavours, smells, temperature and texture of the food.
- Listening to your body's cues of hunger and fullness.

Some people hope that weight loss surgery will take care of their eating and they won't need to think about food anymore. As many of you will know, the opposite is true! To really use your surgery to its maximum potential, you need to eat mindfully and read what your body is telling you, rather than falling into old habits.

To really grasp the concept of mindful eating, it is wise to do further reading from an expert in the field like Michelle May (www.amihungry.com) or Susan Albers (www.eatmindfully.com). Visit their websites to check out some of the great tools they have available.

In the meantime, here are some tips to get you started:

Be Aware

When you are eating, really taste the food and avoid mindless munching. Food provides pleasure and it is important to gain the maximum enjoyment from it each time you eat.

Savour

To get the most out of your eating experience it is important to really experience what the particular food has to offer. Take note of the texture, the smell and the flavour. For example, is it crunchy or smooth, sweet, salty or spicy? Can you tell the different ingredients in the food? Are you really enjoying this food as you eat it?

Avoid Judgment

Food is neither good or bad, it is what we do with it that matters. All food can have a place in our diet, it is the frequency and amounts that are important. Try to avoid labeling food as good or bad and avoid strict food rules. You have the choice to include any food you desire and you have the choice to eat it mindfully and responsibly.

Be in the Moment

Move away from the television or computer. You cannot focus on what you are eating if you are immersed in something else. Avoid playing with your mobile phone or other electronic devices. Avoid eating on the run, or in the car. Choose a relaxing environment to eat. If the staff room at work is too distracting, head outside to a nearby park. Opt for a quiet café rather than a noisy food court, where you may be tempted to rush. Try putting all food on a plate, even snacks, to truly increase your awareness of what you are eating each day.

Be especially careful when eating socially, as during conversation it is very easy to become distracted. Eat during a break in conversation. Avoid the tendency to want to keep pace when eating with others.

Observe

Listen to your body! It provides important cues for when it is time to eat and how much you should eat. If your stomach is rumbling, or you feel genuinely empty or lightheaded, then it is time to eat. When you are eating, pause and see what your body is telling you. Do you feel satisfied? Is the amount you have eaten likely to last you for several hours? Do you need more? Just because you can fit more, does not mean you need it. Overeating after weight loss surgery can cause pain, discomfort, regurgitation and potentially longer term complications.

Take notice when you do slow down your eating and eat more mindfully. Do you feel more satisfied? Do you enjoy your food more? Many people report they enjoy food more after surgery as they eat more slowly, allowing them to really taste the food and savour the flavours.

> "You will enjoy eating more now because you will savour every mouthful and be more selective how you fill the space!"
>
> - Robby, gastric band -

Eat until satisfied

Feeling satisfied and feeling full after eating are not the same. To eat until satisfied means to eat until you are no longer hungry. Eating until full can cause some discomfort, indicating you have eaten too much. Continuing to eat too much over a long period of time will compromise your weight loss.

Eating until satisfied will guide the amount of food you should be eating. Whilst serving sizes are recommended throughout this book, you need to listen to your internal cues to judge how much to eat.

People who have dieted for many years may have lost touch with the signals they get when eating. It is important to re-learn how to listen to your body's signals to judge how much to eat.

Eating mindfully, as has just been discussed, is the first step in allowing you to tune in to your internal cues. The following scale is also useful to help you understand your internal signals and when is the right time to eat and to stop eating.

> "There have been numerous changes but the biggest has been my relationship with food - learning to understand nutrition rich small serves is all I need. I am OK with leaving food now, I do not need to finish my plate."
> - Sharon, gastric bypass -

> "It's not a matter of seeing how much you can eat and get away with, but how little you can eat and be satisfied."
> - Dr Teresa Girolamo, Bariatric GP -

HUNGER AND SATIETY SCALE

Don't get to this point - you risk making poor food choices or eating too quickly

Aim to eat here

Stop eating here!!

Don't eat until this point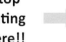

1. Starving, ravenous. All you can think about is how hungry you are.

2. You may have a headache or feel weak or grumpy.

3. You feel like it's time to eat.

4. Your hunger is just starting, but you could wait to eat. Your stomach is starting to feel empty.

5. Neutral. Not hungry, not full.

6. Satisfied or "just right". You are no longer hungry, but probably will be in about three or four hours.

7. You had a few bites too many. You are a little uncomfortable.

8. Full. You definitely don't need more food.

9. Your stomach feels stuffed, uncomfortably full.

10. Painful. So full you feel like you could vomit.

Cut food into small pieces

Cutting food into small pieces makes it easier to chew properly and reduces the risk of discomfort and/or blockages. Many people report not being able to tolerate particular foods after weight loss surgery. This may not be the fault of the food but the size of the pieces they are trying to swallow. Cutting food into very small pieces is even more important if you have dentures or are missing teeth, particularly your back molars.

In the first three to six months after surgery, try to cut all food to the size of a five cent piece. Over time you may find you can manage slightly larger bites, closer to the size of a ten cent piece, but as your bites get bigger always ensure you are chewing well. Never let your bite sizes creep up to the size of a 50 cent piece.

Avoid situations where you are likely to take large bites. Avoid getting really hungry. The hungrier you are when you start a meal, the more likely you are to eat quickly, take big bites and not chew properly. Avoid eating on the run, or in the car, where you will not be focused on your bite size. Avoid eating with your hands, as you will tend to take bigger bites. Always try to sit at a table and use cutlery.

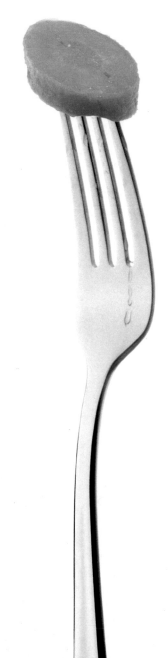

"I now cut my crumpet into 8 pieces; I used to cut it into 2."

- Graham, gastric band -

Chew thoroughly

When food is not chewed properly before swallowing it may cause discomfort and/or blockages.

Helen Bauzon is a consultant bariatric dietitian and author of *The Gastric Band Nutrition Essential and Weight Loss Surgery Nutrition Shopping Guide*. She describes a method of chewing that has helped her patients improve their chewing technique. This technique is beneficial after all forms of weight loss surgery, not only gastric banding. In summary, it includes the following steps:

1. Don't push food straight to the side of your mouth to begin chewing as soon as it enters your mouth. Place the food on your tongue and move it around to experience the textures and flavours.
2. When saliva starts to flow and lubricate the food, move it to the side of your mouth and begin chewing.
3. Bring the food back to your tongue and experience the change in taste and texture.
4. Swallow.

Helen has found this technique extremely successful in helping her patients tolerate a variety of foods. If you are unable to chew food to a smooth texture or crumb in the mouth, avoid eating it. For example, avoid tough, chewy or doughy food.

Choose solid food and avoid liquid calories

In general, solid food tends to empty more slowly from a stomach than liquid, helping us to feel satisfied for longer after eating. For example, you are more likely to feel satisfied for longer after eating roast chicken and vegetables than you are after a chicken and vegetable soup. Chewing helps send signals to your brain that you are eating, helping you feel satisfied. It is important to drink enough fluid to keep hydrated, but once you have recovered and progressed past the fluid diet, it is best to focus on solid food for your meals.

Whilst keeping hydrated is important, the type of fluid is important to ensure you don't take in too many calories or kilojoules.

Avoid regular cordial, soft drinks, full cream milk, milkshakes, smoothies, flavoured coffee, energy and sports drinks and flavoured water. Whilst juices contain some vitamins and minerals, they are high in natural sugar and should be limited.

Water is the best drink. Low or reduced fat milk is fine in small amounts and can help you to achieve two to three serves of milk and milk products daily. A skinny latte, cappuccino or flat white is fine to include as part of your allowance of milk products.

Whilst diet or no sugar forms of carbonated drinks are available, they may cause discomfort after weight loss surgery. The gas in fizzy drinks can cause discomfort in some people. It is best to avoid fizzy drinks in the recovery period after surgery. Before you experiment with fizzy drinks, wait until you feel completely recovered. Discuss in more detail with your surgeon or dietitian.

To keep hydrated, try to drink at least 1500mL (1½L) of fluid each day. If you are not drinking with meals, you must remember to drink regularly throughout the day to meet this target.

> "Soft drinks don't work for me, they bubble up in my tummy."
>
> *- Denise, gastric bypass -*

To snack or not to snack?

People are often told to avoid snacking after weight loss surgery for fear it will slow weight loss. Certainly, eating when you are not hungry (non hungry eating) and grazing can hinder your weight loss potential. If you are tuned in to your hunger signals and making smart snack choices, snacking may be fine.

It is not healthy to snack just because:

- You are bored, tired, happy, angry, sad, etc.
- The clock says it is morning or afternoon tea time.
- Other people are eating.
- You are finishing snacks the children haven't eaten.
- Your partner/housemate/colleague/family like to snack.
- You are in a particular situation eg. you always have to get an ice cream at the beach, popcorn at the movies, lollies on long car trips, chips watching the TV.

It is fine to have a small snack between meals if you are genuinely, physically hungry. It may be that your body needs more food than the basic three meals per day. Or it may be that you can only eat very small meals and need some small snacks to meet your nutritional needs. However, in some cases it may be that your food choices at meals are not satisfying you.

If you find you need to snack, ask yourself the following:

- Are you eating regular meals?
- Are your meals made up of solid foods or are they sloppy food or liquids that may not be satisfying you?
- Are you actually thirsty, rather than hungry?
- Are you eating enough protein containing food at each meal?
- Are you choosing low GI foods (low glycemic index foods)?

If you are physically hungry, a small, healthy snack is acceptable. Focus on nutritious snacks – when you are eating small amounts, try to make every mouthful count. Take the opportunity between meals to eat the food items that you are missing out on at meal times due to your smaller stomach capacity.

The most satisfying snacks are those containing some protein and low GI carbohydrate. Some snacks will contain both and these are the best choice. Some will only offer one of these and are a good choice.

Snacks containing protein and low GI carbohydrate:

- Slice of toasted or plain raisin bread or fruit loaf topped with ricotta cheese or Philadelphia® Extra Light (trim crusts if needed).
- Yoghurt, particularly Chobani® yoghurts as these are higher in protein.
- Low fat yoghurt and fruit.
- Homemade ice block made with pureed fruit and yoghurt such as Chobani®.
- Home made smoothie, milkshake or milk coffee made with low or reduced fat milk. To boost the protein you can add whey protein isolate powder or use higher protein milk such as The Complete Dairy™ milk.
- Skinny cappuccino, latte or flat white.
- Wholemeal/wholegrain crackers eg. Ryvita® or Vita-Weat® with low fat cottage cheese, reduced fat grated cheese, tuna or salmon, hommus, tzatziki or avocado smash (avocado, feta, lemon and cracked pepper).
- Mini can of baked beans.
- A small handful of nuts, seeds and dried fruit (30-50g).
- Protein balls (page 109).

- Dates filled with nut paste.

Snacks containing protein only:

- Hard boiled egg
- Small tin of tuna/salmon
- Slice of cheese
- Small handful of nuts (30-50g)
- Celery or carrot sticks with nut paste.

Snacks containing low GI carbohydrate only:

- Slice of toasted or plain raisin bread or fruit loaf with a scrape of margarine (trim crusts if needed).
- Half a toasted wholegrain English muffin with 100% fruit spread.
- Piece of fruit eg. apple, pear, banana, apricots, plum, peach.
- Frozen fruit cut into pieces eg. oranges, bananas, pineapple.
- Homemade ice block made with pureed fruit.
- Ryvita® or Vita-Weat® with sliced tomato/ avocado.

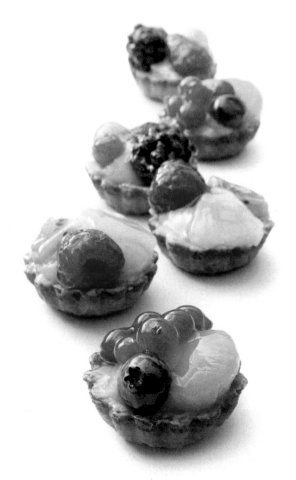

"I freeze yoghurts so they are like ice cream to boost my calcium intake."

- Lisi, gastric bypass -

Protein Balls

These fabulous protein ball recipes are courtesy of Kylie, who had sleeve gastrectomy surgery in 2013. Kylie lost over 35kg to become a healthy weight and this experience ignited her passion for healthy food, wellness and helping others navigate the minefield of post weight loss surgery life.

Method for all Protein Balls

Add nuts to a food processor and process until they form a nut meal. Add the rest of the dry ingredients. Slowly add water (or lemon juice in the Lemon protein balls) until the mixture is moist enough to form balls. Be sure to add the water very slowly as it is easy to add too much which will make the mixture sloppy. Roll into 12 balls.

Choc Cashew Protein Balls

Makes 12 balls

100g cashews

50g almonds

80g whey protein isolate powder

35g shredded coconut

2 tablespoons cocoa

4 medjool dates

Water to bind

Nutrition information (per ball): energy 610kJ, calories 146, protein 9g, fat 8.5g, saturated fat 2.5g, carbohydrate 8g, fibre 1g.

Lemon & Coconut Protein Balls

Makes 12 balls

150g almonds

80g whey protein isolate powder

35g shredded coconut

4 medjool dates

Juice of 2 lemons, approximately 100ml

Nutrition information (per ball): energy 610kJ, calories 146, protein 9g, fat 9g, saturated fat 2g, carbohydrate 7g, fibre negligible.

Choc Hazelnut Protein Balls

Makes 12 balls

150g hazelnuts

35g coconut

6 medjool dates

80g whey protein isolate powder

2-3 tablespoons cocoa

Water to bind

1 hazelnut for the center of each ball

Once you have rolled these ingredients into balls as per the previous method, push one whole hazelnut into the centre of each ball.

Nutrition information (per ball): energy 735kJ, calories 175, protein 9g, fat 11g, saturated fat 2.5g, carbohydrate 10g, fibre negligible.

Pistachio, Cranberry & Chocolate Protein Balls

Makes 12 balls

60g pistachios

90g almonds

80g cranberries

35g coconut

80g whey protein isolate powder

2-3 tablespoons cocoa

Water to bind

Nutrition information (per ball): energy 595kJ, calories 142, protein 9g, fat 9g, saturated fat 2.5g, carbohydrate 6g, fibre 1g.

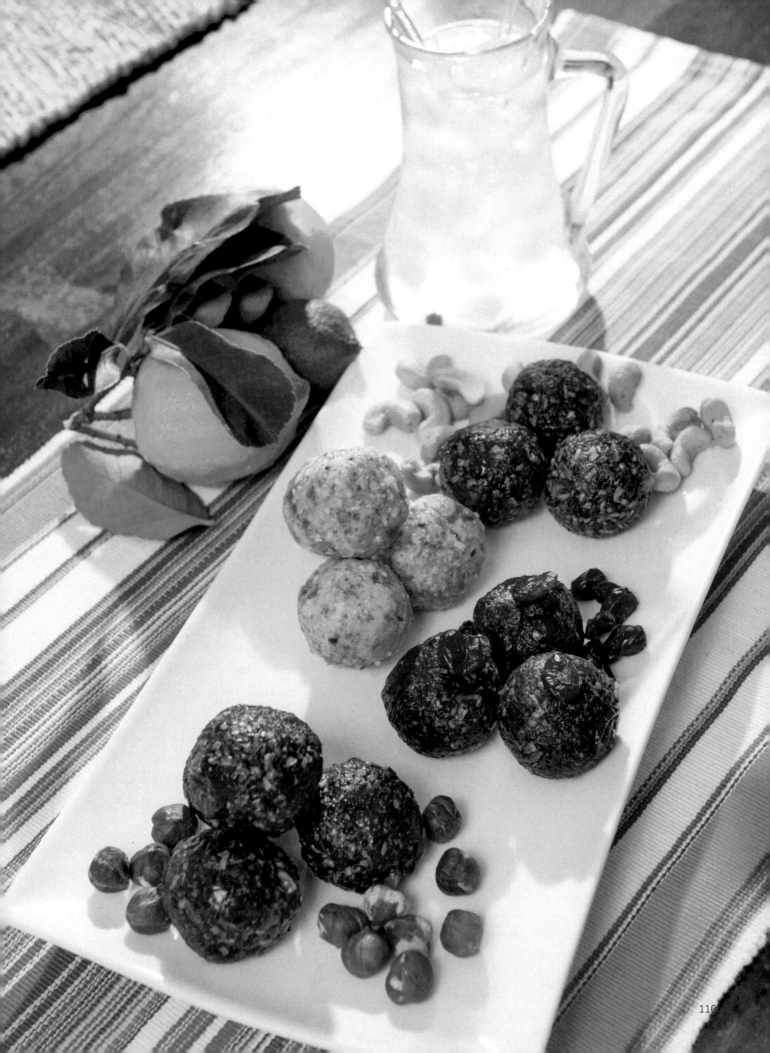

Indulge occasionally

Indulgences or extras are high in energy (calories or kilojoules) and provide little of the vitamins and minerals we need, for example deep fried foods, cake, doughnuts, chocolate, biscuits, chips, pies, pasties, lollies, processed meat, soft drink and pizza.

These foods are not 'bad' foods - they are simply 'occasional' foods. No food is good or bad, it is how we use it and the portions that we eat it in that is important.

Including these foods on a regular basis can lead to an excess energy (calorie or kilojoule) intake and prevent you from achieving your weight loss goals. They can also replace more nutritious foods in your diet, making it hard for you to get all the nutrients you need for good health.

However, it is not reasonable to tell yourself to never eat these foods. The more you tell yourself you must never eat something, the more you will want it. Healthy living is about balance. Indulge in something you enjoy occasionally.

> "I am able to embrace 'SOMETIMES FOOD' thinking. I find that special foods are even more enjoyable than ever because I take the time to eat it slowly, savor it, and eat guilt free."
> - Robby, gastric band -

> "I eat like I am French, I eat everything I want, but I eat in small portions."
> - Tania, gastric bypass -

Alcohol

Alcoholic drinks are generally high in energy (calories or kilojoules). They can increase your appetite and alter your judgment around food, making it difficult to manage your weight.

Alcohol in moderation is not harmful, but an excessive alcohol intake can lead to health problems. The National Health and Medical Research Council (NHMRC) recommend that men and women include no more than two standard drinks per day.

A standard drink is often less than most people consume, particularly those poured at home.

The following is equal to one standard drink:

- 285ml full strength beer (which is less than one can or stubby)
- 30ml spirits
- 100ml white wine, red wine or champagne.

It is important to note however that for people who have had gastric bypass or sleeve gastrectomy surgeries, the absorption of alcohol is changed because an enzyme in the stomach which usually begins to digest alcohol is absent or greatly reduced. Following these surgeries, alcohol may also be absorbed more quickly into the body and this absorbed alcohol will be more potent. Studies have shown these people reach a higher blood alcohol level and maintain this level for a longer time than others. For these reasons, it is wise to drink alcohol cautiously after bariatric surgery. It is even more important not to plan to drive if you are drinking.

Whilst in general there are some reported health benefits of alcohol consumption, it is not recommended that non-drinkers start to drink alcohol for this reason. If you enjoy alcohol, consider it an 'indulgence' and incorporate it into your life as such.

Good Nutrition

The *Food Fundamentals* chapter is not complete without a general discussion on good nutrition and how the recipes in this book have been designed to provide you with a balanced intake.

A balanced intake

Food is made up of combinations of protein, fat and carbohydrate, which all supply the body with energy (calories or kilojoules).

Some foods are higher in one of the particular nutrients and are often referred to in this way, as indicated below.

Carbohydrate-containing Foods

- breads
- cereals
- pasta
- rice
- noodles
- potato
- sweet potato
- corn
- fruit
- fruit juice
- milk
- yoghurt
- foods containing flour
- foods containing sugar (natural or added)

Protein-containing Foods

- meat
- chicken
- fish
- seafood
- eggs
- milk
- milk products
- tofu
- legumes
- nuts

Fat-containing Foods

- oil
- butter
- margarine spreads
- cream
- sour cream
- fatty meat
- full cream milk products

Throughout the book you will find sample menus for each of the dietary stages. These are designed to give you a balance of protein, fat and carbohydrate. However, the menus are only suggestions. People have different tastes and preferences and not everyone will like all of the recipes. It is fine to mix and match the recipes to create a menu you enjoy, but try to keep in mind that a balance of protein, carbohydrate and fat is important. For example, it would not be balanced to have cereal for breakfast, pasta salad for lunch and pasta for dinner every day; just as it would not be balanced to have eggs for breakfast, omelette for lunch and meat for dinner. Ensure you mix and match a variety of foods from all food groups.

In the early stages following sleeve gastrectomy and gastric bypass you will be eating such small serves that it is difficult to get the full range of nutrients for good health. Work closely with your dietitian to maximise your intake at all stages of your journey.

Recipe ingredients

The ingredients in the recipes have been selected for a particular reason. These are discussed below.

Protein-containing foods

Lean protein foods are used in recipes, as they are lower in fat, particularly saturated fat. Meat should be trimmed of fat and chicken should have skin removed. Low fat milk, yoghurt and reduced fat cheeses are recommended.

Protein helps you feel satisfied for longer after eating, making it a very handy nutrient when trying to manage your weight. For this reason the recipes throughout the book were developed to maximise protein intake. Further, when you sit down to a meal, eat the protein-containing foods first.

For more on protein, see the *Nutritional Impacts of Weight Loss Surgery and Supplementation* (page 232).

Fat-containing foods

There are three basic types of fat and each has a different effect on the body.

Saturated fats increase the level of total cholesterol and 'bad' cholesterol (LDL) in our body. They are also associated with other harmful effects in the body; for example, they may increase the risk of cancer. Whilst many people may argue otherwise and you are bound to encounter many opinions, the overwhelming body of evidence and expert opinion (from appropriately qualified experts) is that people generally need to eat less of this type of fat.

Saturated fats are found in:

- meat fat and chicken skin
- full cream cow's milk, cheeses, yoghurts and ice cream
- butter, lard and dripping
- unspecified oils, blended vegetable oil and palm oil
- coconut oil, coconut milk and coconut cream.

Foods high in saturated fat were avoided in the recipes in this book.

Monounsaturated and polyunsaturated fats help reduce the level of bad cholesterol (LDL) in the blood. These are the fats that should be included in the diet.

Unsaturated oils are found in:

- plant oils (except palm and coconut oils)

- seeds
- nuts
- fatty fish
- avocados
- olives
- nut pastes.

Due to the beneficial type of fat in fish, the Heart Foundation suggests you include fish two to three times a week. There are lots of recipes containing fish to choose from in this book to help you meet this target.

Some recipes recommend a particular type of oil be used due to the flavour of that oil. Where a recipe simply states 'oil' or 'oil spray', choose unsaturated oils, such as:

- olive oil
- canola oil
- peanut oil
- rice bran oil
- sesame oil
- soybean oil
- sunflower oil.

Carbohydrate-containing foods and the glycemic index

Where possible, higher fibre and/or low glycemic index (GI) carbohydrate-containing foods were used in the recipes.

The GI is a measure of the effect that different carbohydrate-containing foods have on blood glucose (blood sugar) levels. It describes the way our body digests and absorbs these foods.

Some carbohydrate-containing foods are broken down and absorbed quickly, so they raise our blood glucose level faster and higher. These are high GI foods. Other carbohydrate-containing foods are digested and absorbed more gradually, causing a slower, longer lasting rise in blood glucose levels. These are low GI foods. Low GI foods keep us feeling satisfied for longer after eating.

Research has shown that people eating a lower GI diet can reduce their average blood glucose levels, which is particularly important for people with diabetes. A lower GI eating pattern also helps us feel satisfied for longer after eating, which can help with losing weight.

Foods are classified as low, moderate or high GI. To follow a low GI diet, try to choose one low GI food at each meal. Eat high GI foods in small amounts, or less often.

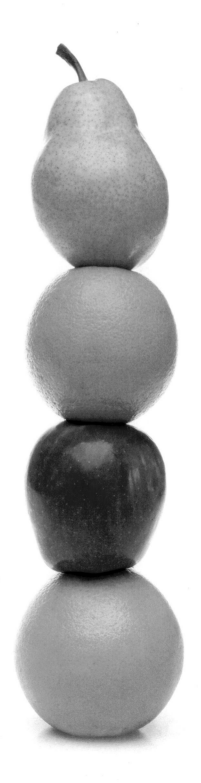

LOW GI	MODERATE GI	HIGH GI

Breads

LOW GI	MODERATE GI	HIGH GI
• wholegrain/multigrain breads • soy and linseed bread • fruit loaf/raisin bread	• wholemeal bread • crumpets • pita bread • rye bread	• white bread • bagels • baguettes • English muffins

Cereal and Grain Foods

LOW GI	MODERATE GI	HIGH GI
• pearl barley • pasta (white or wholemeal) • Doongara® Clever Rice® • Mahatma® rice • fresh rice noodles • semolina • quinoa	• Basmati rice • wild rice • dried rice noodles • cous cous • popcorn	• Jasmine rice

Breakfast Cereals

LOW GI	MODERATE GI	HIGH GI
• porridge • All-Bran® (all varieties) • Guardian® • Sustain® • rice or oat bran	• Weetbix® • Vita-brits® • natural muesli • Mini-wheats® (plain) • Just Right® • Special K®	• Rice Bubbles® • sultana bran • cornflakes • bran flakes • puffed wheat • Coco Pops® • Mini-wheats® (fruit)

Crackers

LOW GI	MODERATE GI	HIGH GI
• Ryvita® Pumpkin Seeds & Oats • Ryvita® Sunflower Seeds & Oats	• Ryvita® original	• water crackers • rice cakes • rice crackers • Corn Thins® • Sao®

Milk and Milk Products

LOW GI	MODERATE GI	HIGH GI
• milk or soy milk • yoghurt		

LOW GI	MODERATE GI	HIGH GI

Fruit

• apple	• rockmelon	• watermelon
• apricot	• pineapple	
• banana	• cherries	
• grapes	• sultanas	
• orange	• raisins	
• peach	• dried fig	
• pear	• fresh paw paw	
• kiwi fruit		
• mango		
• plum		
• prunes		
• dried apricot		
• dried apple		

Vegetables

• sweet corn	• sweet potato	• most other potatoes
• Carisma® potatoes	• broad beans	
• lentils		
• chick peas		
• split peas		
• kidney, soya, baked beans		

Go to www.glycemicindex.com for further information.

Sugar

Sugar is a form of carbohydrate. We tend to get plenty of sugar naturally in fruit and milk products without needing to add it to the foods and drinks we eat. Sugar is rarely added to recipes throughout the book. If it is, it is in very small quantities and the purpose is to enhance a particular flavour.

Salt

A high salt intake is one factor thought to be involved in developing high blood pressure. Salt is made up of sodium and chloride. Some sodium is needed to help maintain the right balance of fluid in our bodies; however we tend to get enough salt from a healthy diet, without having to add it.

As many obese people have high blood pressure, it is useful to limit salt intake to manage this. For this reason, salt reduced and no added salt products are recommended in the recipes.

Energy

'Energy' comes from the food that we eat and is measured in calories or kilojoules (kJ). Food is made up of lots of different nutrients. As discussed earlier, carbohydrate, protein and fat provide energy in foods. Alcohol also provides energy. Water, vitamins, minerals and fibre provide no energy.

Our weight depends on the amount of energy we take in and the amount we burn up. If we take in more energy than we burn, we gain weight. If we eat less energy than we burn, the body will use the excess it has stored and we will lose weight.

There is no exact recommended energy intake for people who have had weight loss surgery, just as there is no single recommended energy intake for people who have not had surgery.

The recipes are designed to provide a low energy diet with maximum nutrition. Just as is the case before surgery, some people can eat more than others following surgery. That is why no exact serve sizes are recommended. As the recipes make four cups, you can use a one cup serve to estimate whether you need more or less than one cup. Recipes can then be adapted to make the right amount. You can also then discuss the amount you are eating with your surgical team at your next appointment with them.

Recipe analysis

All recipes in this book have been analysed using Foodworks®, a dietary analysis program dietitians use to analyse food intakes and menus. You must remember that analysis can only provide an estimate – the Foodworks® program is very comprehensive, but the food supply changes so regularly that no analysis program could ever be 100% accurate.

All nutrition information is given to the nearest five kilojoules and the nearest calorie. Protein, fat, carbohydrate and fibre content are given to the nearest half of a gram (0.5g).

Recipes for Healthy Living

Using the Recipes for Healthy Living

Serving sizes

The recipes are designed to make approximately four, one cup serves. One cup is roughly the amount that will fill the inside rim of a bread and butter plate.

In the first year following sleeve gastrectomy and gastric bypass surgery, you may only tolerate half a cup at a time. Over time you may be able to eat one cup comfortably.

Following gastric band surgery, some may only tolerate half a cup at a time, others may tolerate one cup. Everyone has a different journey and will tolerate different amounts. Your surgical team will guide you.

Regardless of the surgery you have had, eat slowly and stop before you feel any discomfort.

Tips are included for increasing the serve sizes for families and friends. If you find the suggested serve size is not enough to satisfy you, use the tips for family and friends.

Some of the recipes are suitable to freeze and this is indicated where appropriate.

Throughout the *Recipes for Healthy Living*, recipes suitable for the soft diet are indicated with the S icon.

To maximise your protein intake, when you sit down to a meal, always eat the protein-containing foods first.

Diabetes management

People with diabetes should include at least one serve of a carbohydrate-containing food at each meal. If a recipe does not contain a serve of carbohydrate, a note will be included on modifying the recipe so it is appropriate. If you have diabetes,

discuss your carbohydrate requirement with your dietitian, particularly if you are taking medication or insulin.

Hints and tips

Throughout the recipes, practical hints and tips are included between the yellow lines.

> "Your food is so good!"
> *- Christina, gastric band -*
>
> "Your recipes are easy to prepare, quick to make and delicious to eat. I find that the meals fill you up and I would rather eat these than buy takeaway. Before buying your book I would buy takeaway or just cook high calorie foods. I have now learned to cook with so many new and interesting flavours I hardly ever cook from any other cook books. My favorite recipes would be Chicken Curry, Middle Eastern Lamb, Banana & Cinnamon Wraps and Chicken Schnitzel."
> *- Lisa, gastric band -*
>
> "The recipes in this book are fantastic, it's on the kitchen bench full time."
> *- Paul, gastric band -*
>
> "Your book has been wonderful, it's covered in food scraps!"
> *- Jenny, gastric band -*
>
> "My housemate has been cooking from your book since I had surgery - she's lost 4kg in the last 4 weeks. My sister is a home ec teacher and she's been using the recipes too."
> *- Amy, gastric band -*
>
> "You will still be able to make lovely meals for dinner parties and your family. It is just a matter of portion size and choosing the healthier option."
> *- Dana, gastric band -*

HEALTHY LIVING SAMPLE MENU

Breakfast Options

- Egg with the Lot (page 123)
- Quinoa Porridge with Cinnamon & Berries (page 124)
- Baked Bean Cups (page 125)
- Bircher Muesli (page 126)
- Bacon & Egg Breakfast Muffins (page 127)
- Eggs with Prosciutto in Mushrooms (page 128)
- Nutty Banana & Date Muffins (page 129)
- Nutty Chia Porridge (page 130)
- Muesli (page 131)
- Poached Egg Muffins (page 132)
- Protein Packed Yoghurt, Fruit & Nuts (page 133)
- Sardines with Lemon (page 134)
- Mushroom, Rocket & Tomato Omelette (page 135)
- Peach & Ricotta Muffins (page 136)

Lunch Options

- Pumpkin & Spinach Frittata (page 59)
- Chunky Winter Soup (page 140)
- Asparagus, Quinoa & Feta Salad (page 141)
- Roasted Vegetable & Haloumi Salad (page 142)
- Prawn Laksa (page 143)
- Beetroot, Bean & Feta Salad (page 144)
- Pasta Salad (page 145)
- Pumpkin, Tomato & Chickpea Salad (page 146)
- Tuna & Sweet Potato Frittatas (page 147)
- Tuna & Broccoli Salad (page 148)
- Zucchini Slice (page 149)
- Tuna Niçoise Salad (page 150)
- Tandoori Chicken Salad (page 151)
- Taco Muffins (page 152)
- Roasted Capsicum, Corn & Feta Savoury Muffins (page 153)
- A range of cracker toppings & wrap fillings are provided on pages 155 - 158.

- Oriental Beef (page 161)
- Chicken Stir-fry with Pine Nuts & Raisins (page 162)
- Mexican Fish Parcels with Spicy Mexican Salad (page 163)
- Fajitas (page 165)
- Pork Chow Mein (page 167)
- Chicken Kebabs (page 168)
- Chilli, Ginger & Lime Chicken (page 169)
- Zesty Tomato Fish (page 171)
- Lamb & Rosemary Kebabs (page 173)
- Prawn Paella (page 175)
- Baked Salmon & Cauliflower Puree (page 177)
- Bean & Vegetable Hot Pot (page 178)
- Spicy Barbeque Fish Wraps (page 179)
- Stuffed Capsicums (page 180)
- Meatballs with Vegetable Sauce (page 181)
- Vietnamese Beef & Mint Salad (page 183)
- Middle Eastern Lamb (page 185)
- Beef in Red Wine (page 186)
- Creamy Vegetable Curry (page 187)
- Tasty Tomato Beef (page 189)
- Chicken Creole (page 191)
- Chicken Schnitzel & Chips (page 193)
- Pumpkin, Spinach & Ricotta Cannelloni (page 195)
- Mixed Vegetable Pizza (page 196)
- Chicken Curry (page 197)
- Caesar Salad (page 199)
- Tofu Stir-fry (page 201)
- Veal Parmigiana (page 202)
- Thai Fish Parcels & Stir-fry Vegetables (page 203)
- Chicken Satay Cups (page 205)
- Italian Chicken Pasta (page 206)
- Slow Cooked Lamb Curry (page 207)
- Creamy Chicken & Sweet Potato Casserole (page 209)
- Veal Saltimbocca (page 211)

Breakfast

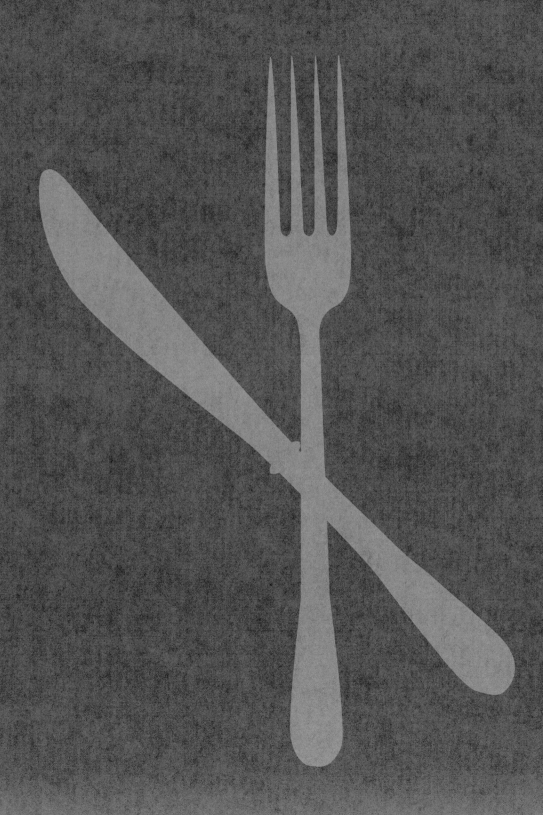

Egg with the Lot

Makes 4 cups

Oil spray

1 cup cherry tomatoes, halved

4 eggs

Pinch of basil

¼ onion, grated

2 bacon eyes, trimmed of fat, finely diced

2 wholegrain/multigrain English muffins

1 cup baby spinach

Freshly ground black pepper

Heat a frying pan that has been sprayed with oil. Add cherry tomatoes and cook until softened. Remove from pan, set aside. Spray 4 egg rings with oil and place in the pan. Beat the eggs, add basil, onion and bacon. Pour the mixture evenly between the egg rings. Cover frying pan and using very gentle heat cook until each of the eggs has set. Split and toast 2 English muffins. Top each muffin half with some baby spinach, cooked egg and cooked tomatoes. Season with pepper to taste.

Nutrition information: kilojoules 825, calories 197, protein 15g, fat 9g, saturated fat 2.5g, carbohydrate 13g, fibre 2.5g.

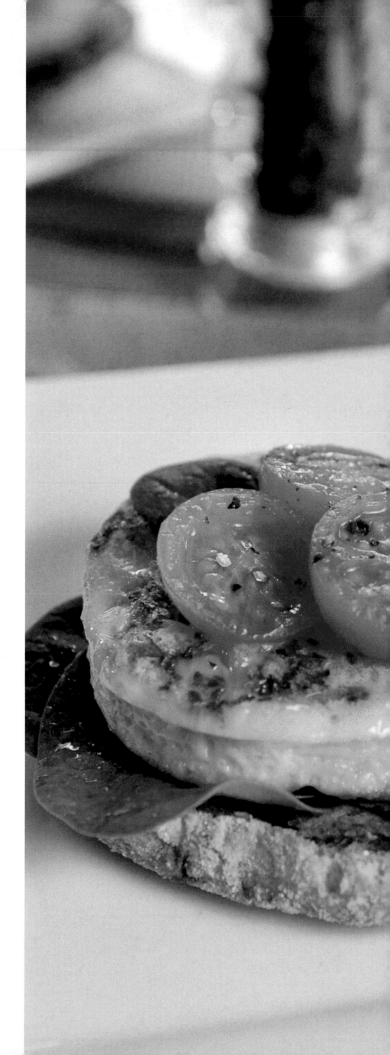

Quinoa Porridge with Cinnamon & Berries S

Makes 4 cups

½ cup quinoa

1¼ cups low or reduced fat milk

½ cup water

1 cup frozen mixed berries, thawed

1 cup Chobani® vanilla yoghurt

2 tablespoons chia seeds

2 tablespoons (30g) whey protein isolate powder

1-2 teaspoons cinnamon (optional)

Combine quinoa, water and 1 cup of the milk in a saucepan and bring to the boil over high heat. Reduce heat, cover and simmer 10 to 15 minutes or until most of the liquid is absorbed. Turn off the heat and let stand, covered, for 5 minutes. Dissolve the protein powder in the remaining milk. Stir through the berries, chia seeds and yoghurt. Add the dissolved protein powder and stir until combined. Sprinkle with cinnamon to serve (optional).

Nutrition information (per cup): energy 1045kJ, calories 250, protein 21.5g, fat 6.5g, saturated fat 2g, carbohydrate 24.5g, fibre 4.5g.

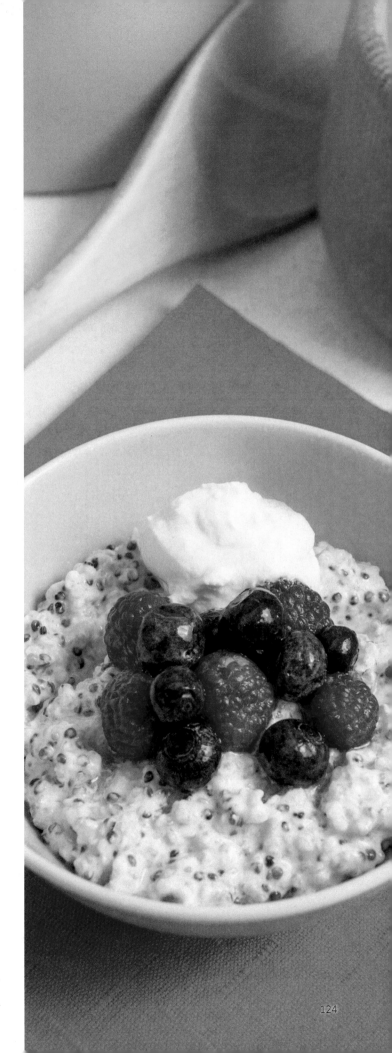

Baked Bean Cups S*

Makes 4 cups

Oil spray

415g can salt reduced baked beans

150g shortcut bacon, trimmed of fat, diced

¼ cup reduced fat grated cheese

2 slices mountain bread

Freshly ground black pepper

Preheat oven to 180°C. Heat a small frying pan that has been sprayed with oil. Add bacon and cook for a couple of minutes. Drain excess fluid from baked beans. Combine beans and bacon. Trim mountain bread pieces so that they will push into 4 cups of a muffin tray and overhang slightly. Divide bean and bacon mixture between muffin cups and bake for 10 minutes. Sprinkle with cheese to serve.

Nutrition information (per cup): kilojoules 1005, calories 240, protein 20.5g, fat 8g, saturated fat 3g, carbohydrate 19.5g, fibre 5g.

S* Baked beans are suitable on the soft diet, however serve plain initially.

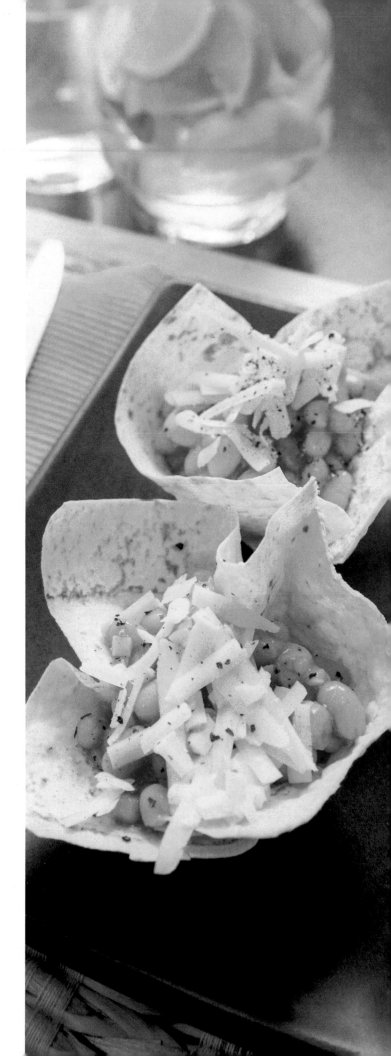

Bircher Muesli S*

Makes 4 cups

1 cup rolled oats

¼ cup hazelnuts, chopped

1 apple, grated

1 cup low fat milk

2 tablespoons sultanas

3 tablespoons (45g) whey protein isolate powder

Sprinkle of cinnamon

Dissolve protein powder in milk. Mix all ingredients until well combined. Leave overnight in refrigerator. When serving, add a little more milk if too stiff.

Nutrition information (per cup): kilojoules 1015, calories 243, protein 16.5g, fat 7.5g, saturated fat 1g, carbohydrate 26g, fibre 3.5g.

S*   Bircher Muesli is suitable on the soft diet, however skip the nuts initially.

Try some flavour variations:

- Serve topped with a dollop of yoghurt and a couple of diced strawberries.
- Hazelnuts can be replaced with almond flakes or slivers, natural or toasted lightly in the oven.
- Sultanas can be replaced with diced dried apricots, apple, pear or raisins.

"I enjoyed this recipe. Half a serve was good for me as I'm new to the sleeve."

- Carmelina, sleeve gastrectomy -

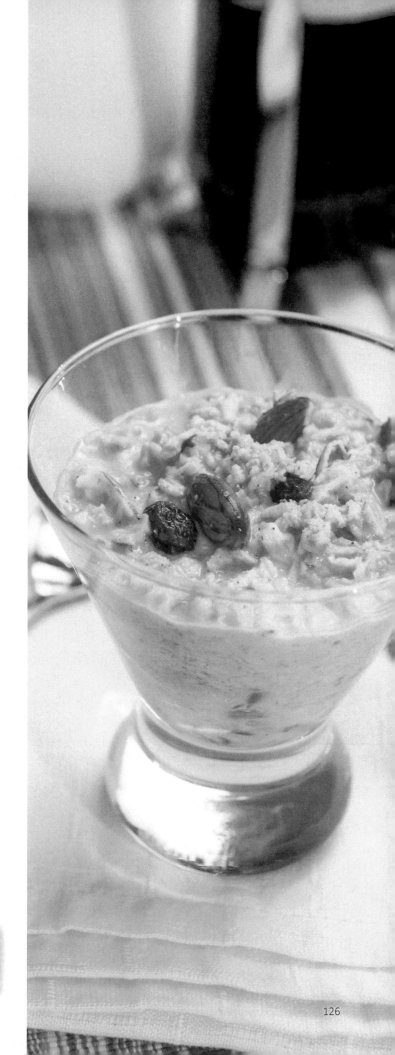

Bacon & Egg Breakfast Muffins

Makes 12 muffins

Oil spray

150g shortcut bacon, trimmed of fat, diced

¼ cup mushrooms, diced

12 eggs

3 spring onions (white part), thinly sliced

1 tomato, diced

¼ cup red capsicum, diced

½ cup baby spinach, shredded

1 cup reduced fat tasty cheese, grated

4 tablespoons whey protein isolate powder

¼ cup low fat milk

Freshly ground black pepper

Preheat oven to 180°C. Line a 12 cup muffin tin with paper liners or spray with cooking spray and set aside. Heat a frying pan that has been sprayed with oil. Add bacon and mushroom and cook gently for a few minutes. In a large bowl, beat eggs. Dissolve whey protein isolate powder in the milk. Add bacon, mushrooms and remaining ingredients and mix well to combine. Scoop ⅓ cup of mixture into each muffin pan. Bake for 20-25 minutes or until the center of the muffin is cooked.

Nutrition information (per muffin): kilojoules 570, calories 136, protein 15.5g, fat 8g, saturated fat 3.5g, carbohydrate 1g, fibre negligible.

Optional: to make Layered Breakfast Muffins, rather than dicing and cooking the bacon, cut it into round pieces, roughly the same size as the bottom of the muffin tray cups (they don't have to be exact). Put two pieces of bacon into each of the holes and bake in the oven for 5 minutes. Follow the rest of the method as per above.

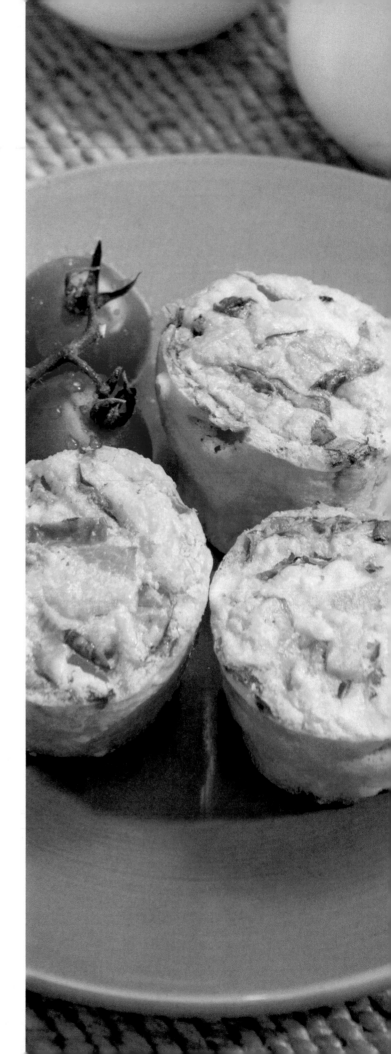

Eggs with Prosciutto in Mushrooms

Makes 4 cups

Oil spray

4 large Swiss brown or Portobello mushrooms (must be 'cup' shaped)

4 slices prosciutto, trimmed of fat

4 eggs

Freshly ground black pepper

Fresh parsley or thyme (optional)

Preheat oven to 180°C. Clean the mushrooms with a damp cloth, remove the stem and scrape out the black gills so you have a 'well' for the egg. Spray the outside of the mushroom with oil. Arrange the mushrooms on a baking tray. Place a slice of prosciutto into each mushroom. Crack the eggs, one at a time, into a small bowl. Carefully slide each egg into a mushroom. Sprinkle with black pepper and parsley or thyme. Carefully place the baking tray into the oven and bake for 20-30 minutes. The amount of time required depends on how thick your mushrooms are and how you like your eggs cooked.

Nutrition information (per cup): energy 740kJ, calories 177, protein 18.5g, fat 9.5g, saturated fat 3g, carbohydrate 2.5g, fibre 4g.

- Prosciutto is quite salty. If you have high blood pressure and need to limit salt, you could replace the prosciutto with fresh spinach leaves.
- If you have diabetes, serve with some wholegrain toast or ½ an English muffin.

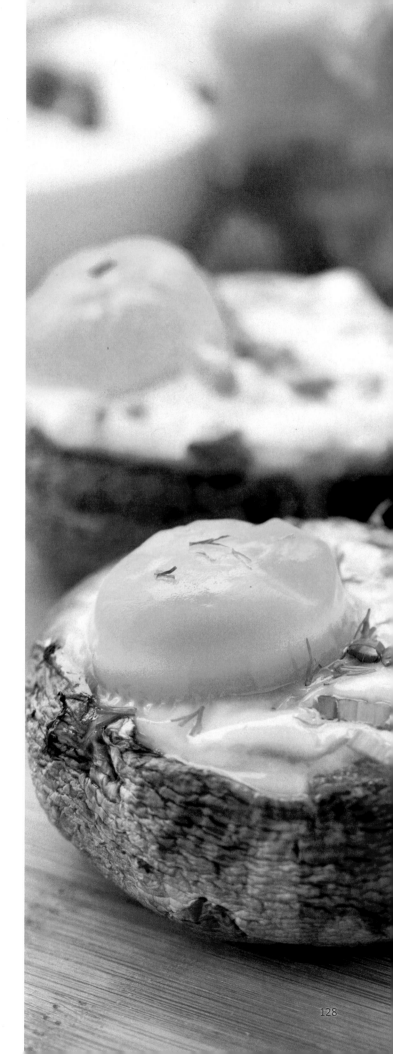

Nutty Banana & Date Muffins

Makes 12 muffins

1 cup wholemeal self raising flour

¼ cup almond meal

¼ cup whey protein isolate powder

¾ cup low or reduced fat milk

1 cup rolled oats

½ cup shredded coconut

2 ripe bananas, mashed

100g medjool dates, chopped

75g flaked almonds

1 egg

Preheat oven to 180°C. Line a 12 cup muffin tin with paper liners or spray with cooking spray and set aside. Dissolve protein powder in ¼ cup of the milk. Combine all ingredients in a bowl and mix until combined. Spoon into the muffin cups and bake until lightly browned on top.

Nutrition information (per muffin): kilojoules 855, calories 205, protein 8g fat 8g, saturated fat 2.5g, carbohydrate 23.5g, fibre 3g.

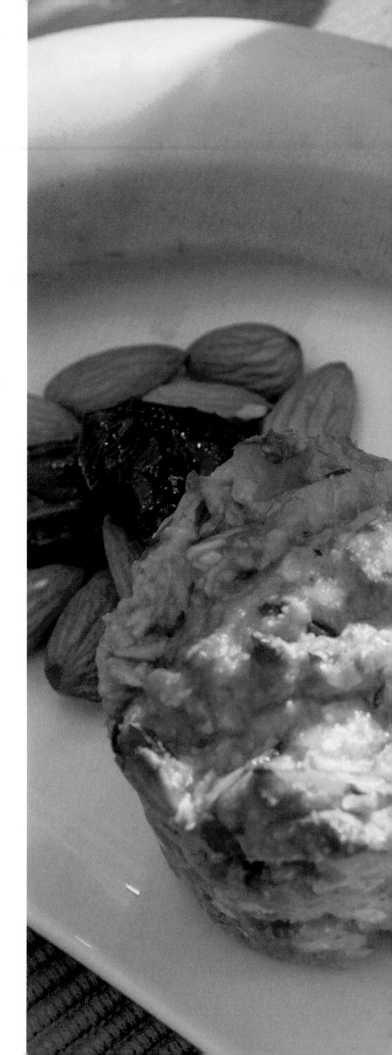

Nutty Chia Porridge 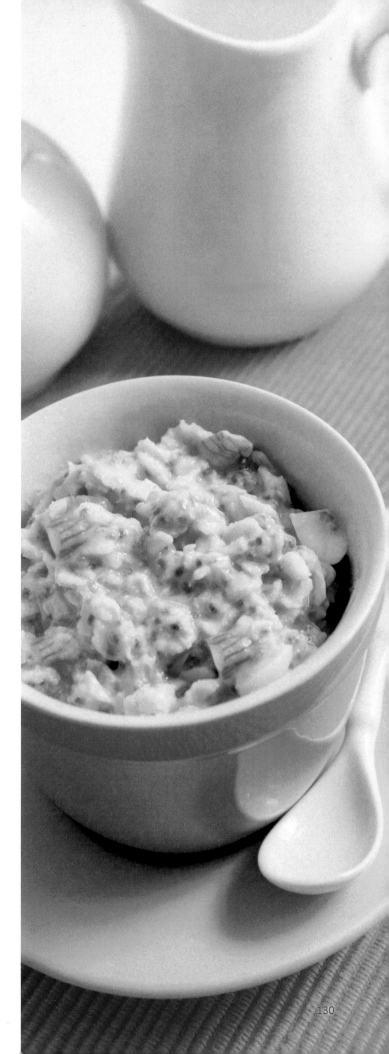 S*

Makes 4 cups

1 cup rolled oats

1 cup low fat milk

¾ cup water

1 tablespoon almond meal

¼ cup almonds, chopped

2 tablespoons chia seeds

1 tablespoon brown sugar

3 tablespoons (45g) whey protein isolate powder

Combine oats, milk and ½ cup of water in a microwave safe container. Cover and microwave for 3 minutes. Stir. If it appears the porridge needs more cooking, microwave for another 1-3 minutes, removing each minute and stirring well. Keep an eye on the porridge as it can easily boil and spill over. Dissolve the protein powder in ¼ cup of water. Stir through almonds, almond meal, chia seeds, brown sugar and dissolved powder. Serve.

Nutrition information (per cup): kilojoules 1190, calories , protein 19g, fat 12.5g, saturated fat 1.5g, carbohydrate 22.5g, fibre 4g.

S* Porridge is suitable on the soft diet, however skip the nuts initially.

Muesli

Makes 4 cups (8 x ½ cup serves)

1½ cups of rolled oats

½ cup of processed bran

½ cup flaked almonds

¼ cup sultanas

¼ cup sunflower seeds

¼ cup pepitas

¼ cup walnuts, broken into smaller pieces

Low or reduced fat milk, to serve

Chobani® yoghurt, to serve

Mix ingredients together and store in an airtight container. Serve ½ cup muesli with a milk and yoghurt.

Nutrition information (per ½ cup serve with milk and yoghurt): kilojoules 940, calories, protein 10g, fat 12g, saturated fat 2g, carbohydrate 19g, fibre 3.5g.

To make toasted muesli, you can simply toast the oats (and nuts and seeds if you wish) before combining with the other ingredients. If using oil spray (which will increase the fat content of the recipe slightly), spread the ingredients out on baking trays and spray with oil. If using apple juice (which will increased the sugar content slightly), combine ingredients in a bowl, add a splash of apple juice and stir well until ingredients are just moist, then spread out on baking trays. Bake in a moderate oven (180°C) for 10-15 minutes, checking regularly to see that you achieve your desired level of toasting.

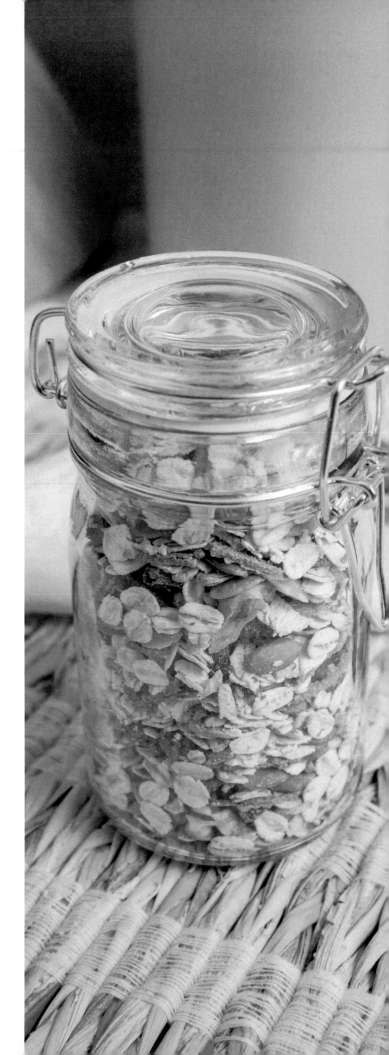

Poached Egg Muffins

Makes 4 cups

2 wholegrain/multigrain English muffins, toasted

2 teaspoons vinegar

4 eggs

2 tomatoes, sliced

Handful of baby spinach leaves, chopped

Freshly ground black pepper

Preheat grill or non-stick frying pan. Add sliced tomato. Cook 5 minutes or as desired. Keep warm. Boil 5cm water in saucepan or frying pan. Add vinegar. Break eggs into a cup, one at a time, and then gently slide each egg into the saucepan. Simmer gently for 2-3 minutes until egg white is set. Top each half of a toasted muffin with baby spinach, grilled tomato and poached egg. Add freshly ground black pepper to taste.

Nutrition information (per cup): kilojoules 645, calories 154, protein 10.5g, fat 6g, saturated fat 2g, carbohydrate 13g, fibre 2.5g.

To prevent the egg white spreading in the water whilst poaching, stir the water in the saucepan until it is spinning like a whirlpool and gently slide an egg into the centre. Eggs will need to be cooked individually using this method.

"Very tasty and refreshing. I found the muffin easy to tolerate, even though I am sometimes wary of bread based products. As an alternative you could add a slice of shaved ham or a sprinkle of spring onion, however it was great as it was."

- Leoni, gastric bypass -

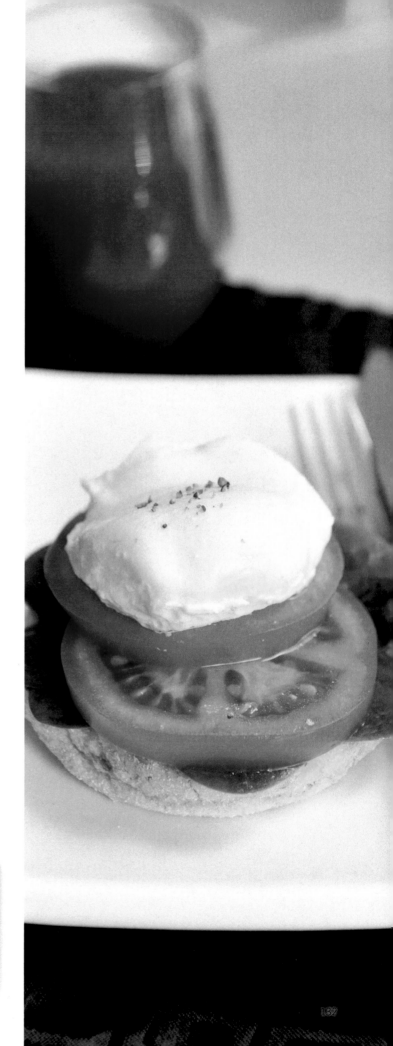

Protein Packed Yoghurt, Fruit & Nuts

Makes 4 cups

1½ cups mixed fruit, diced eg. banana, kiwi fruit, strawberries, rockmelon, passionfruit

2 cups Chobani® low fat yoghurt

2 tablespoons (30g) whey protein isolate powder

½ cup flaked almonds

Sprinkle protein powder into yoghurt and stir until well combined. In 4 small bowls or glasses, layer equal amounts of yoghurt, fruit and flaked almonds.

Nutrition information (per cup): kilojoules 890, calories 213, protein 22g, fat 8.5g, saturated fat 2g, carbohydrate 11.5g, fibre 2g.

We have used Chobani® yoghurt in our recipes as of the commercially available yoghurts, it contains the highest amount of protein. If you like to limit your sugar intake, choose the plain variety. Other brands of yoghurt can be used, however will generally not be as high in protein.

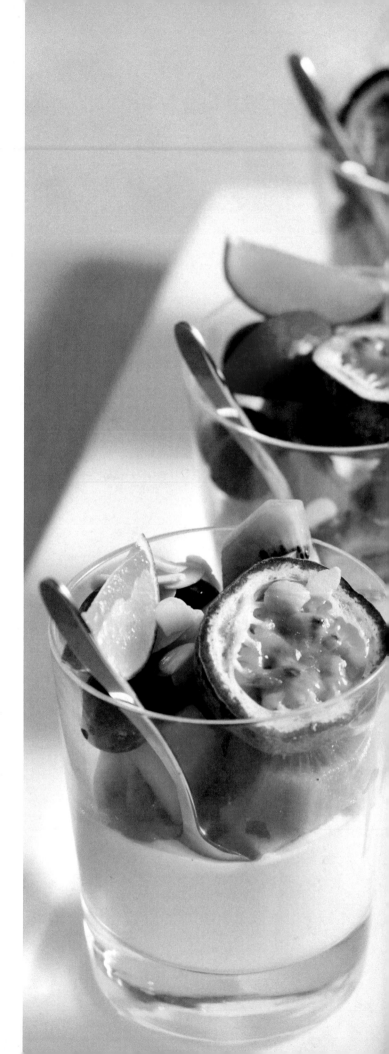

Sardines with Lemon

Make 4 cups

125g can of sardines in water, drained

1 tablespoon of lemon juice

1 spring onion, diced

1 tomato, diced

4 slices wholegrain/multigrain bread

½ cup reduced fat cheese, grated

Freshly ground black pepper

Mash the sardines with the lemon juice, pepper, onion and tomato. Toast bread and spread with the sardine mixture. Sprinkle with cheese and grill, cooking until the cheese is melted. Cut each slice in half and serve.

Nutrition information (per cup): kilojoules 835, calories 200, protein 15g, fat 8g, saturated fat 3g, carbohydrate 16g, fibre 2.5g.

"Yummy!"
- Lyn, gastric band -

"Very filling."
- Jane, gastric bypass -

"This is lovely, just beautiful."
- Elaine, gastric band -

"I can highly recommend the Sardines with Lemon."
- Sonya, gastric band -

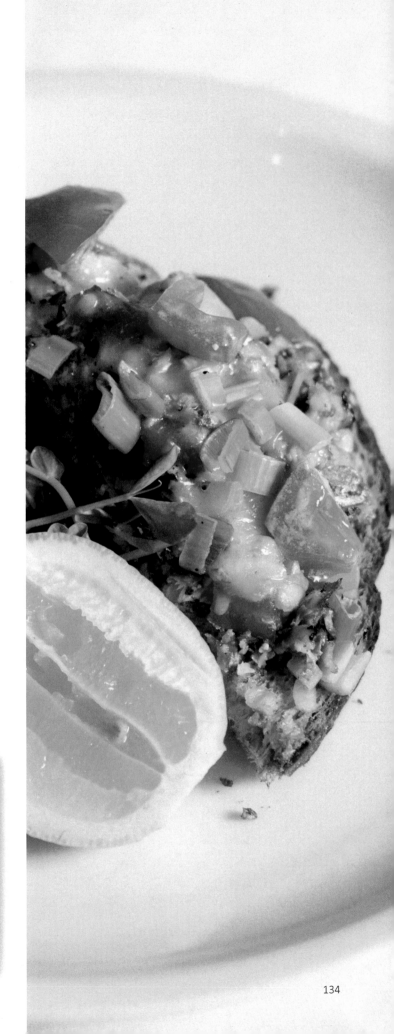

Mushroom, Rocket & Tomato Omelette 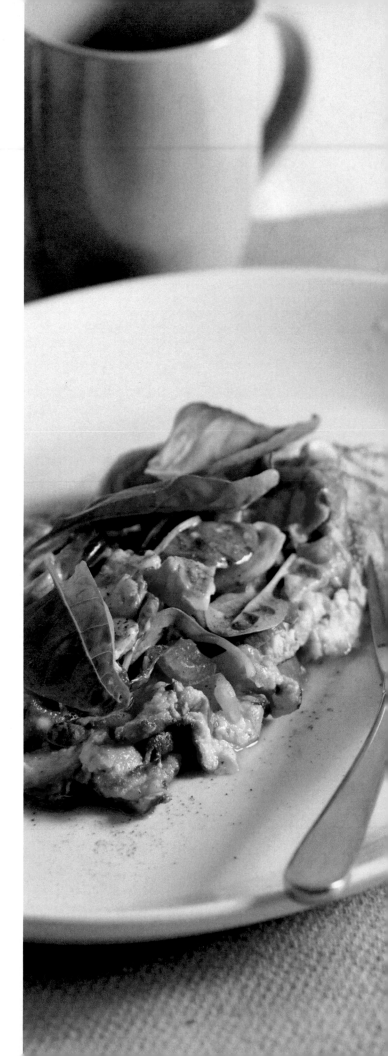 s

Makes 4 cups

Oil spray

8 eggs

2 tablespoons chopped fresh chives

1 cup mushrooms, sliced

1 red onion, finely diced

1 cup rocket or baby spinach, finely chopped

1 cup cherry tomatoes, halved

2 tablespoons Parmesan cheese, grated

Whisk eggs and chives together in a bowl. Set aside. Heat a small frying pan that has been sprayed with oil. Sauté onion and mushrooms until soft. Pour the egg mixture into the hot pan. Cook for 1-2 minutes, or until the underside is firm. Use an egg slice to move the runny top of the mixture underneath to allow all of the mixture to cook. Sprinkle top of omelette with rocket or spinach, tomatoes and Parmesan cheese. Use an egg slice to fold the omelette in half. Serve immediately.

Nutrition information (per cup): kilojoules 800, calories 191, protein 15.5g, fat 12.5g, saturated fat 4g, carbohydrate 3g, fibre 1.5g.

If you have diabetes, have a smaller serve of the omelette with ½ a wholegrain/multigrain English muffin or slice of toast.

Peach & Ricotta Muffins

Makes 4 cups

1 cup low fat ricotta cheese

1/2 cup Chobani® low fat vanilla yoghurt

2 tablespoons (30g) whey protein isolate powder

2 peaches, halved, peeled and sliced

2 wholegrain/multigrain or fruit English muffins, toasted

Cinnamon to serve

Combine ricotta, yoghurt and protein powder and mix well until the mixture is smooth. Grill or barbeque the peach slices until browned on both sides. Halve English muffins and toast. Serve each muffin half topped with the ricotta cheese mixture and peach slices. Sprinkle with cinnamon to taste.

Nutrition information (per cup): kilojoules 1020, calories 244, protein 21g, fat 7g, saturated fat 4g, carbohydrate 22g, fibre 2.5g.

Grilled peaches can be replaced with grilled bananas, nectarines or mango.

"The muffins were really good!!! Easy to make and very tasty!"
- *Sarah, gastric bypass* -

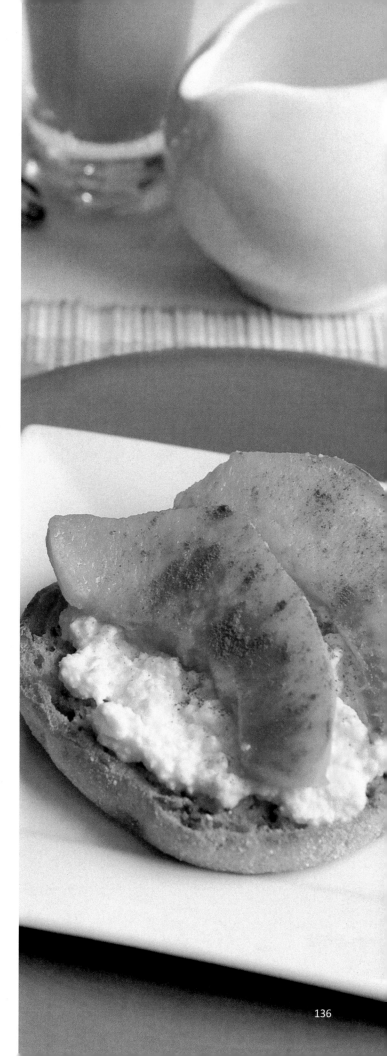

Lunch

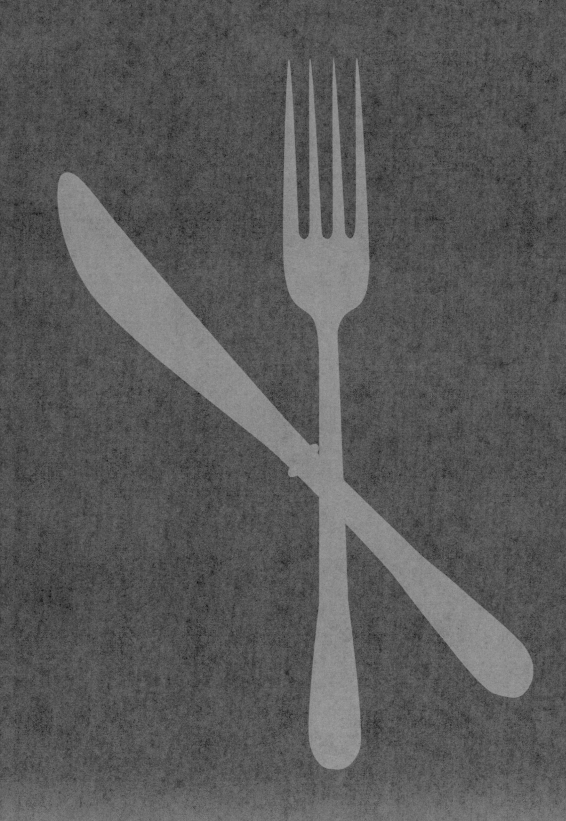

Pumpkin & Spinach Frittata (S)

Makes 4 cups

Oil spray

500g pumpkin, sliced thinly

2 cloves garlic, crushed

1 tablespoon oil

6 eggs

½ cup low fat milk

1½ cups baby spinach

¼ cup Parmesan cheese, finely grated

Pinch of nutmeg

Freshly ground black pepper

Preheat oven to 200°C and spray a baking tray with oil. Place pumpkin slices on a baking tray and roast, uncovered, until the pumpkin is tender. Spray a square cake pan or lasagne dish with oil and line the base and sides with baking paper. Whisk eggs with milk, nutmeg, pepper, garlic and oil. Layer half of the pumpkin in the pan, top with spinach then remaining pumpkin. Pour the egg mixture over the pumpkin and spinach and sprinkle with cheese. Bake, uncovered, for about 25 minutes or until firm. Stand 5 minutes before slicing.

Nutrition information (per cup): kilojoule 1055, calories 253, protein 16g, fat 16g, saturated fat 4.5g, carbohydrate 10.5g, fibre 2g.

- This recipe is included as a suggestion for lunch, as it can be served cold. However, it is also delicious served warm with a side salad as an evening meal.
- Suitable to freeze.

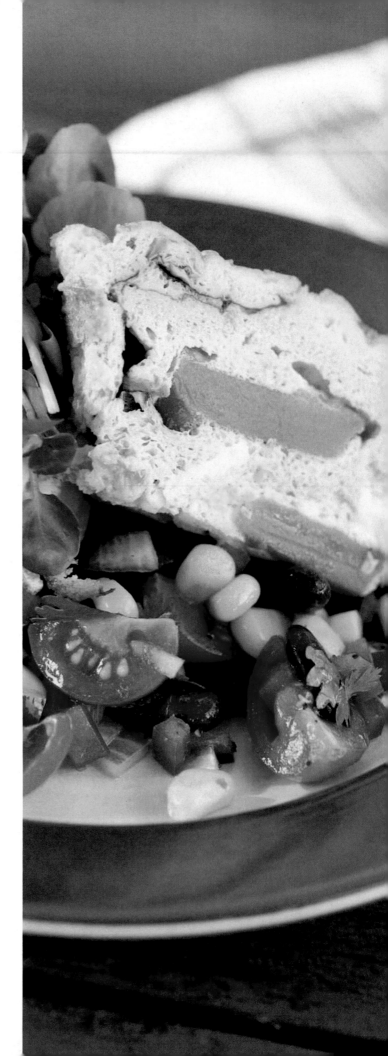

Chunky Winter Soup 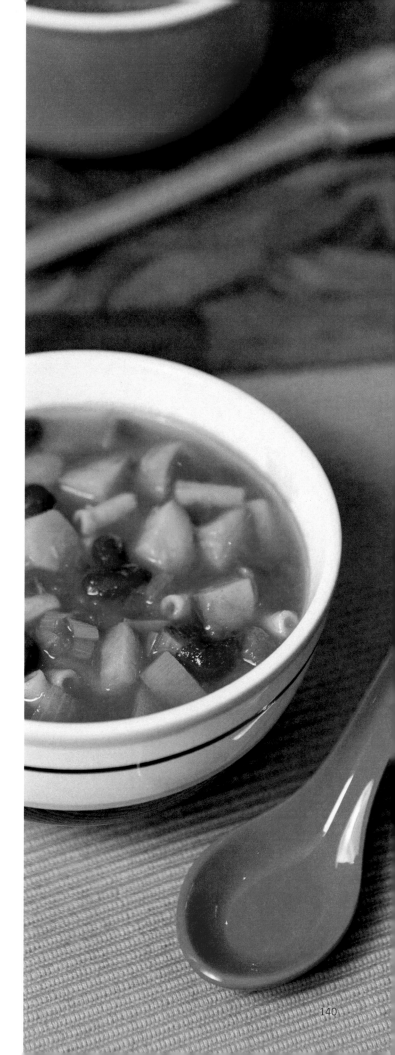 ⓢ

Makes 4 cups

Oil spray

½ onion

1 small or ½ large leek, thinly sliced

2 cups salt reduced chicken stock

1 small or ½ large zucchini, diced

1 small or ½ large carrot, diced

1 cup no added salt, chopped tinned tomatoes

½ teaspoon curry powder

1 tablespoon no added salt tomato paste

Freshly ground black pepper

2 tablespoons macaroni

1 cup cooked red kidney beans

3 tablespoons (45g) whey protein isolate powder

1/4 cup water

Heat a saucepan that has been sprayed with oil. Add onion and leek and cook until they are starting to soften. Add the stock, carrot, zucchini, tomatoes, curry powder, tomato paste and season with pepper. Bring to the boil then simmer for 20 minutes, until vegetables are tender. Add macaroni and kidney beans and simmer for a further 15-20 minutes until the macaroni is cooked. Dissolve protein powder in water and stir through soup.

Nutrition information (per cup): kilojoules 665, calories 159, protein 15.5g, fat 2g, saturated fat negligible, carbohydrate 16g, fibre 6g.

Suitable to freeze. Try freezing in single serves ready to defrost for a quick lunch.

Asparagus, Quinoa & Feta Salad

Makes 4 cups

⅓ cup dry quinoa

¼ cup pepitas

2 spring onions, finely sliced

1 red capsicum, diced

1 bunch asparagus, woody ends removed

¼ cup sundried tomatoes, finely sliced

1 tablespoon red wine vinegar

2 teaspoons olive oil

1/3 cup reduced fat feta, crumbled

Freshly ground black pepper

Place quinoa in a saucepan. Cover with water and bring to the boil. Reduce the heat to low and simmer until quinoa is cooked, approximately 15 minutes. (Quinoa is cooked when fine white rings form around the edge of the quinoa and it is tender to bite.) Drain quinoa and allow to cool in the refrigerator. Preheat grill. Add asparagus and grill until tender. Remove from grill and slice into short lengths. Combine with quinoa and refrigerate. Combine all ingredients and mix well to combine.

Nutrition information (per cup): kilojoules 955, calories 228, protein 12.5g, fat 12g, saturated fat 3.5g, carbohydrate 17g, fibre 4g.

A versatile recipe that works well with some shredded baby spinach and grilled chicken. Family or friends may enjoy these.

"**Very tasty and crunchy, just how I like it. I really liked the red wine vinegar as the dressing - got my tick!**"
- Erica, gastric bypass -

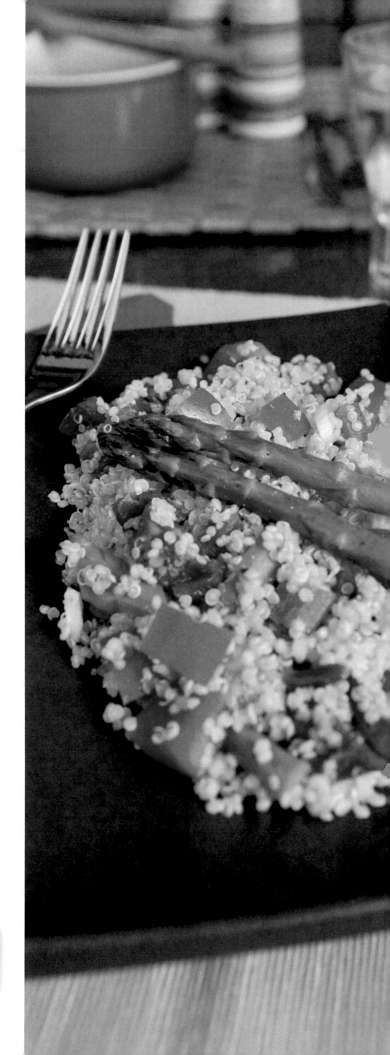

Roasted Vegetable & Haloumi Salad S*

Makes 4 cups

100g haloumi, sliced

½ cup sweet potato, diced

½ red capsicum, sliced

½ zucchini, sliced

1 small carrot, sliced

1 fresh beetroot, sliced

½ onion, sliced

2 cloves garlic, chopped

1 tablespoon fresh rosemary, chopped

1 tablespoon olive oil

½ cup cooked red kidney beans

½ cup cooked chickpeas

1 tablespoon balsamic vinegar

Freshly ground black pepper

Flat leaf parsley, chopped

Combine haloumi, sweet potato, capsicum, zucchini, carrot, beetroot, onion, garlic, rosemary, pepper and oil in a large bowl or freezer bag. Mix until all ingredients are evenly coated with oil. Remove haloumi and fry in a non stick pan for a few minutes either side or until golden. Place vegetables in a single layer in a large baking dish or oven tray. Bake in the oven at 180°C for 35 minutes, or until the vegetables are tender. Stir through kidney beans, chickpeas and vinegar. Garnish with flat leaf parsley.

Nutrition information (per cup): kilojoules 795, calories 191, protein 10.5g, fat 9.5g, saturated fat 3.5g, carbohydrate 13g, fibre 5.5g.

- S* This recipe is suitable on the soft diet if you ensure the vegetables are cooked until tender and can be broken with the side of a fork.
- To boost the protein content a little more, serve with Hummus (page 213).

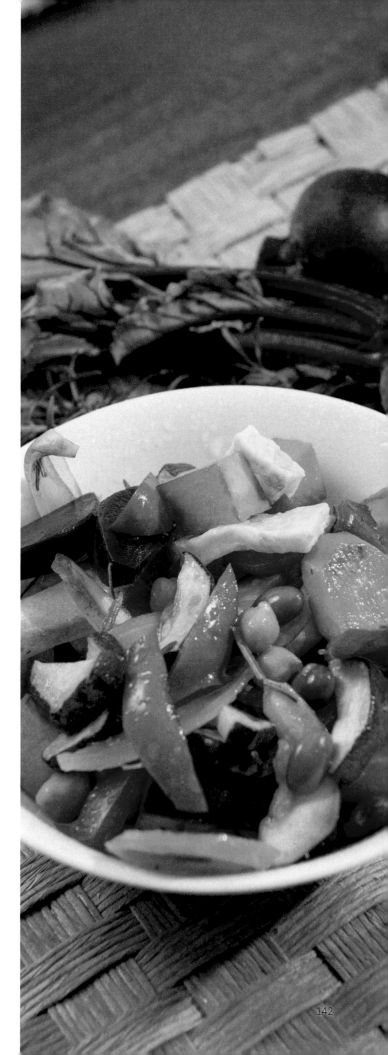

Prawn Laksa

Makes 4 cups

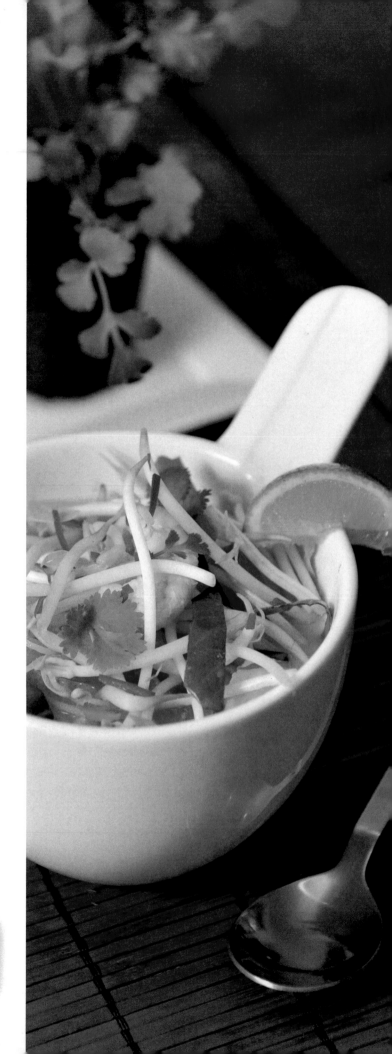

2 tablespoons laksa paste

1½ cups chicken stock

200mL coconut flavoured low fat evaporated milk

¾ cup cold water

40g dried rice vermicelli noodles

250g green prawns

½ red capsicum, sliced into very thin strips

1 bunch bok choy or pak choy, sliced thinly

Bean sprouts, for garnish

Fresh coriander leaves, for garnish

1 red chilli, seeds removed thinly sliced

Lime wedges, to serve

Heat laksa paste in a large saucepan over medium heat for 2 minutes, or until the paste is fragrant. Add stock, evaporated milk and cold water. Cover and bring to the boil. Add noodles, capsicum and bok choy and simmer for 4 minutes or until the noodles are tender. Add prawns and simmer for 2 to 3 minutes or until prawns turn pink. Divide laksa between bowls. Top with bean sprouts, coriander and chilli. Serve with lime wedges.

Nutrition information (per cup): kilojoules 805, calories 193, protein 18.5g, fat 5.5g, saturated fat 1.5, carbohydrate 16.5g, fibre 2g.

Suitable to freeze without garnish. Add these to serve.

"The Prawn Laksa from Sally's book has become my go to recipe"
- Ben, gastric band -

Beetroot, Bean & Feta Salad

Makes 4 cups

1⅓ cups cooked butter beans (or 400g can, drained & rinsed)

450g can tinned beetroot wedges, drained

½ cup reduced fat feta cheese, crumbled

¼ cup loosely packed mint leaves

¼ cup unsweetened apple juice

2 tablespoons mustard

4 tablespoons chopped walnuts

2 handfuls baby spinach leaves

Place apple juice and mustard in a small jar and shake well. Combine beans, beetroot, feta and walnuts in a bowl. Pour over dressing and combine well. Fold through baby spinach to serve.

Nutrition information (per cup): kilojoules 845, calories 202, protein 12.5g, fat 11.5g, saturated fat 3.5g, carbohydrate 10.5g, fibre 5g.

"Yummy! Quick, easy, great for an easy to pack lunch."
- Melissa, sleeve gastrectomy -

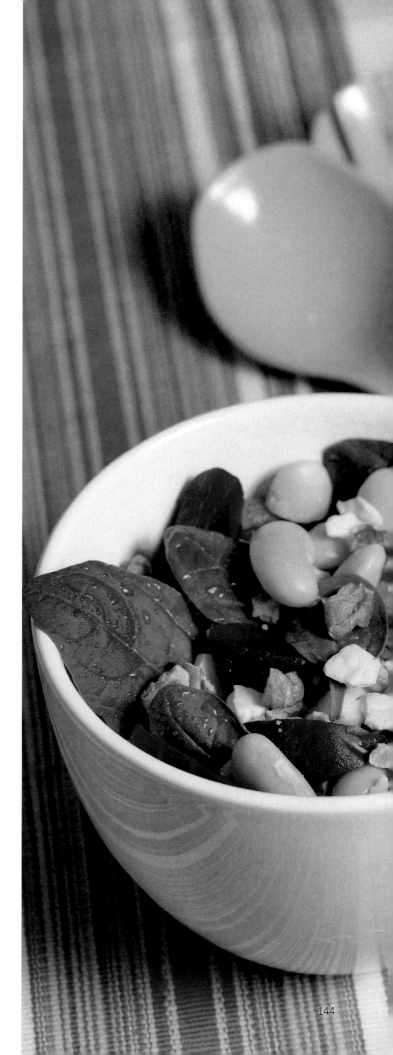

144

Pasta Salad

Makes 4 cups

50g dry pasta eg. spirals

2 x 130g can skinless, boneless salmon in springwater, drained

½ cup sun dried tomatoes, sliced 60g

1 small yellow capsicum, sliced

½ Lebanese cucumber, diced

½ carrot, peeled into ribbons with a potato peeler

Freshly ground black pepper

Dressing

¼ cup low fat natural yoghurt

¼ cup low fat mayonnaise

1 clove garlic, crushed

1 tablespoon lemon juice

1 tablespoon wholegrain mustard

To make dressing, combine all ingredients in a jar and shake to mix. Cook pasta according to packet instructions. Drain and toss in dressing to prevent pasta becoming dry. Stand until thoroughly cool. Mix with remaining ingredients and season with pepper to taste. Refrigerate until required.

Nutrition information (per cup): kilojoules 995, calories 238, protein 19g, fat 8g, saturated fat 12g, carbohydrate 19.5g, fibre 3.5g.

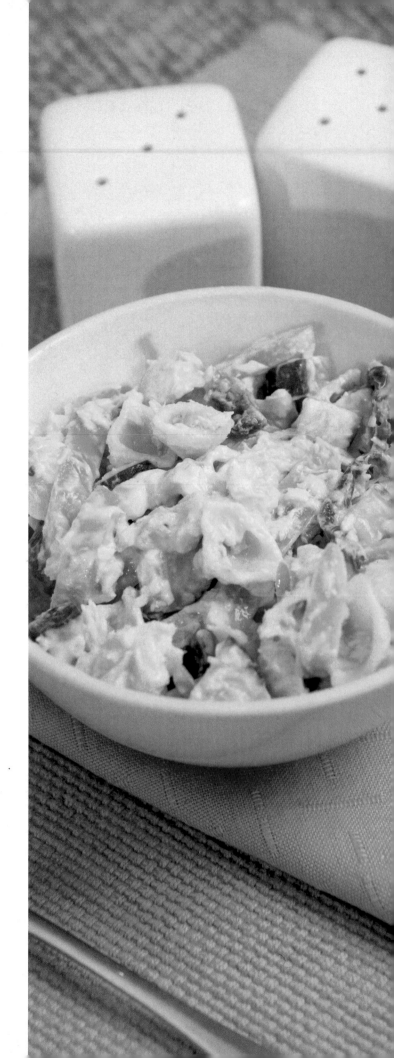

Pumpkin, Tomato & Chickpea Salad

Makes 4 cups

Oil spray

2 cups pumpkin, diced

1½ cups cooked chickpeas (or 400g can chickpeas, drained and rinsed)

1 cup cherry tomatoes, halved

½ cup reduced fat feta, crumbled

1-2 tablespoons fresh coriander (or parsley), finely chopped

Freshly ground black pepper

2 tablespoons pine nuts, toasted

1 tablespoon lemon juice

1 tablespoon balsamic vinegar (optional)

Preheat oven to 200°C. Spray a baking tray with oil. Spread diced pumpkin over tray. Cook for approximately 10-15 minutes or until tender. Remove from oven and allow to cool. Combine all ingredients and mix well.

Nutrition information (per cup): kilojoules 1040, calories 249, protein 16g, fat 12g, saturated fat 4g, carbohydrate 16g, fibre 5.5g.

"Beautiful!"

- Michelle, gastric band -

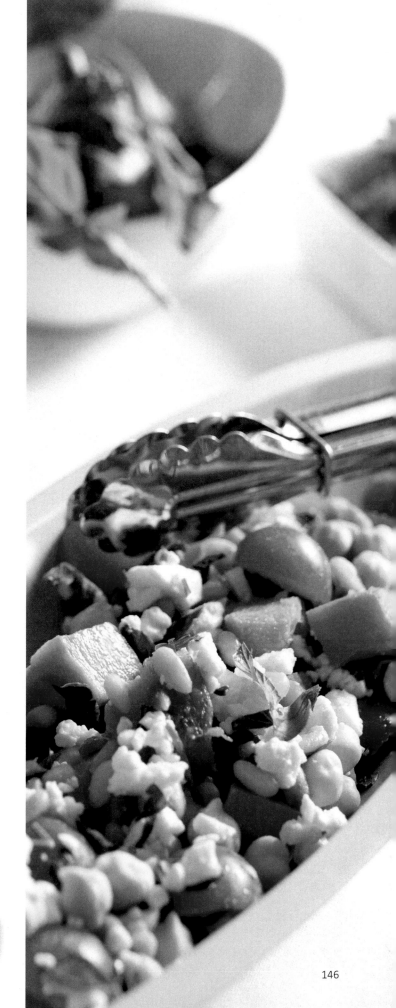

Tuna & Sweet Potato Frittatas ⓢ

Makes 4 cups (8 mini frittatas)

Oil spray

1½ cups sweet potato, peeled and diced into 1cm cubes

5 eggs, lightly whisked

¼ cup low fat milk

185g tuna in spring water, drained well and flaked

125g can corn kernels, drained

½ small red onion, finely diced

1 tablespoon Parmesan cheese, finely grated

2 tablespoons chives, chopped

2 tablespoons oats

Freshly ground black pepper

Pre-heat oven to 180°C. Add the sweet potato to a medium saucepan, cover with cold water, bring to the boil and simmer for 5 minutes or until sweet potato is tender. Drain the sweet potato and set aside to cool a little.

Spray 8 x ½ cup capacity muffin pans with oil spray. Combine the eggs, milk, tuna, corn, onion, Parmesan, chives and oats. Season with black pepper and then add in the sweet potato and stir gently to combine. Spoon this mixture evenly into the muffin pans. Bake for 20-30 minutes or until cooked through (cut into one of the frittatas with a knife - if there is no milky fluid and it is solid it is cooked). Remove from oven and let stand for 15 minutes. Serve warm or cold, with or without salad.

Nutrition information (per cup): kilojoules 970, calories 232, protein 19.5g, fat 9.5g, saturated fat 3g, carbohydrate 16g, fibre 2g.

Suitable to freeze. A great lunchbox option.

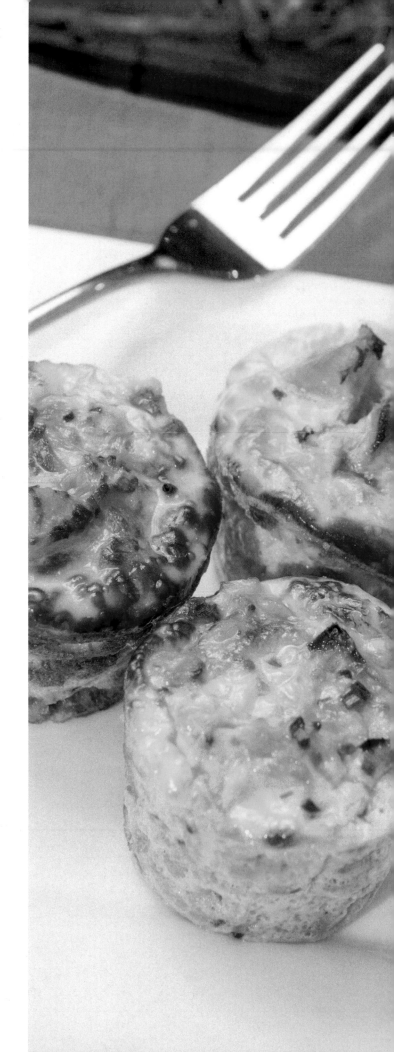

Tuna & Broccoli Salad

Makes 4 cups

2 cups broccoli, cut into small florets

8 snow peas, strings removed

½ cup cherry tomatoes, halved

185g can tuna in spring water, drained

½ cup fresh parsley, chopped

½ yellow capsicum, diced

¼ cup fat free Italian dressing

Fresh herbs to garnish

Boil, steam or microwave broccoli until just tender. Rinse under cold water and drain well.Place snow peas in boiling water until they change colour, approximately 30-60 seconds. Rinse under cold water, drain well and slice into thin slivers. Combine broccoli, snow peas, tomatoes, flaked tuna, parsley, capsicum and dressing in a large serving dish. Drizzle salad dressing over salad and garnish with fresh herbs.

Nutrition information (per cup): kilojoules 370, calories 88, protein 12.5g, fat 1g, saturated fat 0.5g, carbohydrate 5g, fibre 3g.

If you have diabetes, add some croutons made from toasted wholegrain/multigrain bread. Alternatively, include a smaller serve of salad and finish the meal with some fruit.

> **"I love uncooked broccoli - a very tasty salad that I would recommend others to try."**
> *- Erica, gastric bypass -*

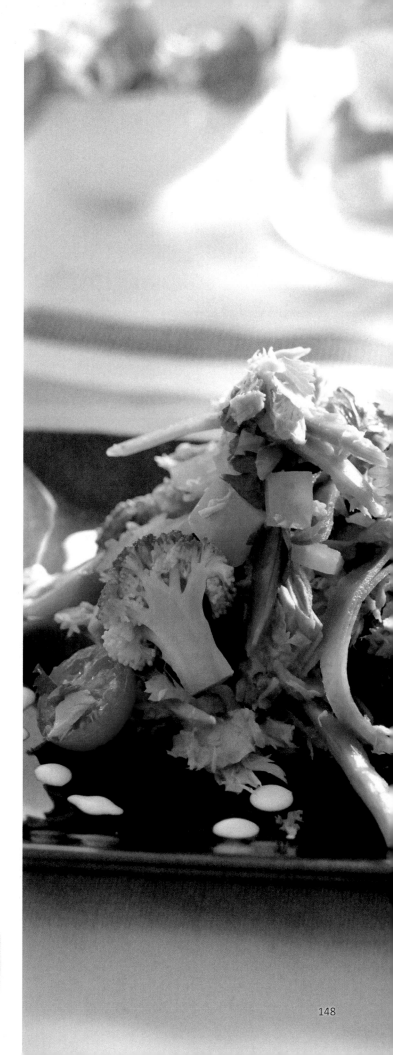

Zucchini Slice S

Makes 4 cups

2 zucchini, grated

1 carrot, grated

½ onion, finely diced

125g tin corn, drained

1 tablespoon sundried tomatoes, diced

2 eyes of bacon, rind removed, finely diced

½ cup reduced fat tasty cheese, grated

⅓ cup white self-raising flour

⅓ cup wholemeal self-raising flour

4 eggs

1 tablespoon reduced fat feta, crumbled

Freshly ground black pepper, to taste

Sprinkle of basil and thyme

Preheat oven to 200°C. Combine zucchini, carrot, onion, bacon, corn, sun dried tomatoes, cheese, sifted flour and lightly beaten eggs. Season with pepper and a sprinkle of basil and thyme. Line a lamington or cake tin with baking paper. Pour mixture into the tin and bake for 30-40 minutes or until browned.

Nutrition information (per cup): kilojoules 1140, calories 273, protein 20g, fat 12g, saturated fat 5g, carbohydrate 19g, fibre 3.5g.

- For lots of flavour with little fat, choose sundried tomatoes vacuum packed with little oil.
- Suitable to freeze. Freeze in single serves for a quick and easy lunch.

"This is great. I haven't baked in 20 years. The whole family love it. It's great after footy training for my son."
- Sarah, gastric band -

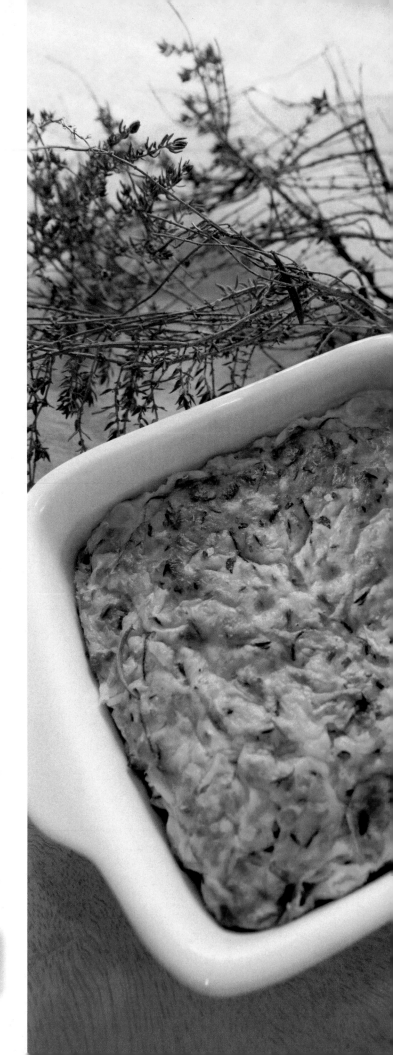

Tuna Niçoise Salad

Makes 4 cups

200g green beans, topped, tailed and cut in half

2 tomatoes, each cut into 8 wedges

2 hard-boiled eggs, halved

185g can tuna in spring water, drained

12 black olives

¼ cup low fat mayonnaise eg. Kraft Free®

2 teaspoons French mustard

Lettuce, to serve

Place beans in a heat proof container. Boil kettle and pour boiling water over beans to cover. Leave for a few minutes, until beans are bright green. Drain and refresh in cold water. Drain again. Combine tuna with mayonnaise and mustard and mix well. Combine beans, tomato, eggs, tuna mixture and olives. Serve with lettuce.

Nutrition information (per cup): kilojoules 655, calories 157, protein 15g, fat 6g, saturated fat 1.5g, carbohydrate 8.5g, fibre 3g.

If you have diabetes, add some croutons made from toasted wholegrain/multigrain bread. Alternatively, include a smaller serve of salad and finish the meal with some fruit.

> **"This is an excellent reworking of a traditional Niçoise salad. All the flavour and texture, minus the fat."**
> *- Robyn, gastric bypass -*
>
> **"Delicious.'**
> *- Lyn, gastric band -*

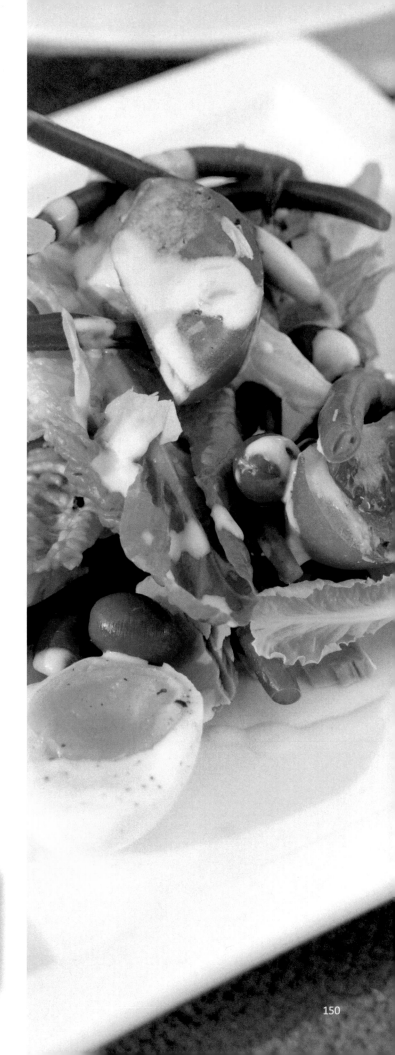

Tandoori Chicken Salad

Makes 4 cups

Oil spray

400g skinless chicken, trimmed of fat, cut into strips
eg. breast, tenderloin or thigh

1 tablespoon Tandoori paste

1 Lebanese cucumber, cut into thin slices

1 cup snow peas, strings removed

½ cup low fat tzatziki (see *Ingredients* page 213)

Few handfuls baby spinach leaves

Lemon wedges, to serve

Combine chicken with Tandoori paste and mix well
until chicken is well coated with paste. Heat a frying
pan that has been sprayed with oil. Add chicken and
cook until it is cooked through. Combine cucumber,
snow peas and baby spinach in a bowl. Divide salad
between serving plates, top with chicken pieces and
tzatziki and serve with lemon wedges.

Nutrition information (per cup): kilojoules 910, calories 218, protein 23g,
fat 11.5g, saturated fat 3g, carbohydrate 4.5g, fibre 2g.

- The tzatziki recipe makes a great dip for
  when you have guests, or use as a spread for
  sandwiches, crackers or wraps.
- If you have diabetes, serve with some mini
  pappadums cooked in the microwave.

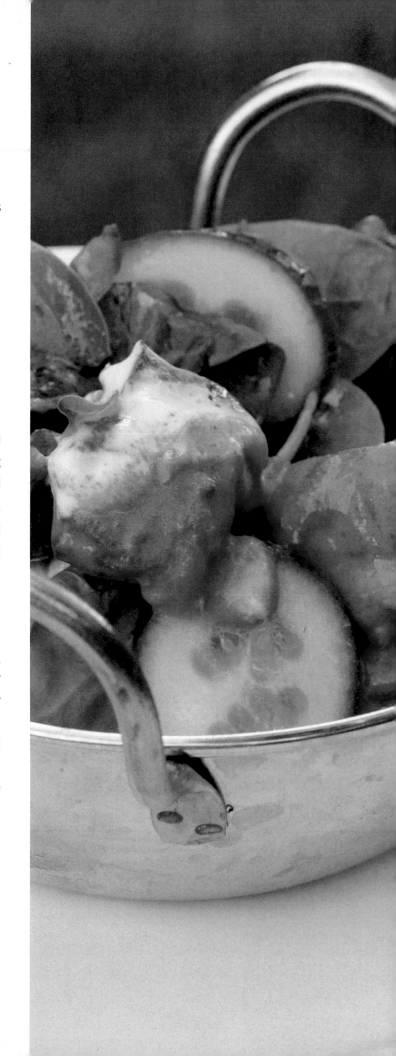

Taco Muffins

Makes 12 muffins

250g lean beef mince

2 tablespoons taco seasoning

1/3 cup water

12 eggs, lightly beaten

425g can kidney beans, drained

425g can diced tomatoes

½ green capsicum, diced

½ onion, diced

1 cup reduced fat tasty cheese, grated

Optional: salsa, natural yogurt and avocado,
to taste

Preheat oven to 180°C. Line a 12 cup muffin tin with paper liners or spray with cooking spray and set aside. Heat a frying pan that has been sprayed with oil. Add the mince and cook for a few minutes or until slightly browned. Stir in the water and taco seasoning and cook for another two or three minutes. Lightly whisk the eggs in a large bowl. Stir in the mince, beans, tomatoes, capsicum, onion and cheese. Spoon into the muffin tin and bake for approximately 25 minutes or until cooked.

Optional: Serve with salsa, natural yogurt or diced/mashed avocado if desired.

Nutrition information (per muffin): kilojoules 670, calories 160, protein 15.5g, fat 8.5g, saturated fat 4g, carbohydrate 5.5g, fibre 2.5g.

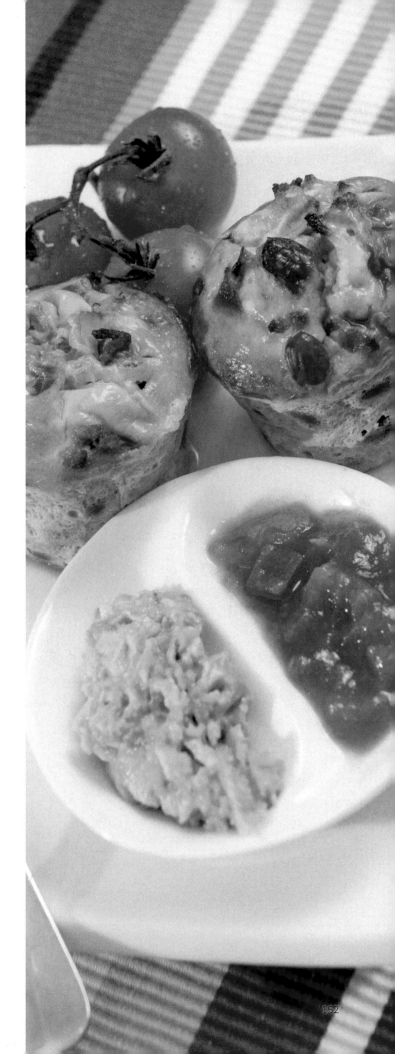

Roasted Capsicum, Corn & Feta Savoury Muffins

Makes 12 muffins

1 zucchini, grated

125g tin corn, drained

½ cup roasted capsicum, diced 60g

½ cup reduced fat tasty cheese, grated

½ cup reduced fat feta, crumbled

½ cup white self raising flour

½ cup wholemeal self raising flour

6 eggs

2 tablespoons chives, chopped

4 tablespoons whey protein isolate powder

¼ cup low or reduced fat milk

Freshly ground black pepper, to taste

Preheat oven to 200°C. Line a 12 cup muffin tin with paper liners or spray with cooking spray and set aside. Combine zucchini, corn, capsicum, cheeses, sifted flour and lightly beaten eggs. Dissolve protein powder in milk and stir through the mixture. Season with pepper and a sprinkle of chives. Pour mixture into the muffin pans and bake for 20-25 minutes or until the center of the muffin is cooked.

Nutrition information (per muffin): kilojoules 680, calories 163, protein 15g, fat 6.5g, saturated fat 3.5g, carbohydrate 11g, fibre 1.5g.

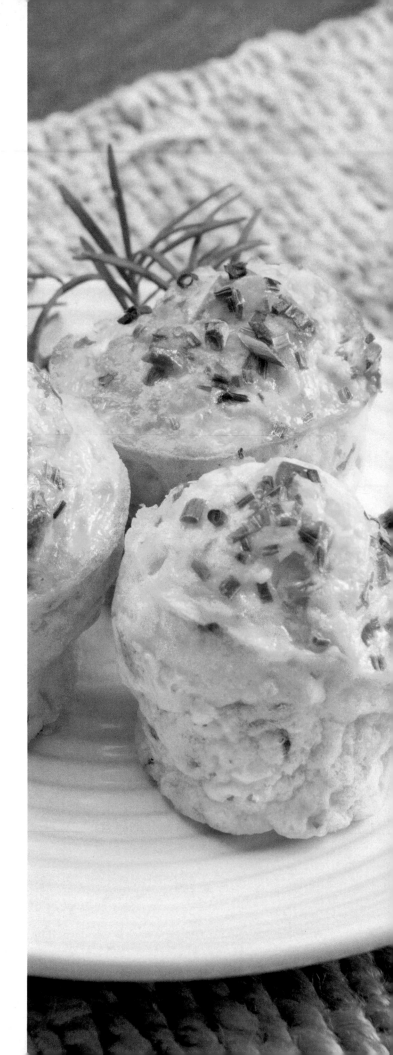

Cracker Toppings & Wrap Fillings

Mexican Crackers

Makes 4 cups

½ cup cooked kidney beans

½ tomato, diced

¼ cup tomato salsa

2 tablespoons corn

½ medium carrot, grated

¼ cup reduced fat tasty cheese, grated

½ avocado

8 Ryvita® crackers or 4 Vita-Weat® Lunch Slices

Combine all ingredients except avocado and crackers. Mix well. Spread crackers with avocado. Top with combined mixture.

Nutrition information (per cup): kilojoules 840, calories 201, protein 7g, fat 9.5g, saturated fat 2.5g, carbohydrate 19g, fibre 6g.

- This recipe works well as a wrap. Add finely chopped baby spinach and roll up firmly in 4 slices of wholemeal or rye mountain bread.
- The toppings and fillings for crackers, pita bread and wraps can be swapped for different bases. If you tolerate bread, choose the grainy varieties and use the fillings for a regular, open, or toasted sandwich. Experiment with different bases and fillings to make lunch most satisfying for you.

Roasted Vegetable & Hummus Pita

Makes 4 cups

2 teaspoons olive oil

1 tablespoon lemon juice

2 wholemeal pita bread

½ medium zucchini

½ large red capsicum (or 1 small)

½ large eggplant (or 1 small)

4 heaped tablespoons hummus (see *Ingredients* page 213)

1 cup packed baby spinach, rocket, or finely shredded lettuce

Freshly ground black pepper

Preheat oven to 200°C. Thinly slice all vegetables and then further slice into strips. Toss vegetables in oil and lemon juice, season with pepper. Place on a baking tray and cook in the oven for approximately 20 minutes or until cooked. Cut each pita in half to make 2 smaller pockets. Spread hummus on one inner side of the pocket. Stuff each pocket with vegetables and baby spinach.

Nutrition information (per cup): kilojoules 710, calories 170, protein 6g, fat 7.5g, saturated fat 1g, carbohydrate 17g, fibre 5g.

Salmon on Crackers

Makes 4 cups

425g tin salmon in spring water, drained

1 tablespoon fresh chives or dill, chopped (or 2 teaspoons minced chives or dill)

2 tablespoons low fat mayonnaise eg. Kraft Free®

2 tablespoons lemon juice

½ cup cucumber, finely sliced

½ avocado, sliced

Freshly ground black pepper (optional)

8 Ryvita® crackers or 4 Vita-Weat® Lunch Slices

Flake salmon with a fork and mix with chives, mayonnaise and lemon juice. Top crackers with cucumber and avocado then spread with salmon mixture.

Nutrition information (per cup): kilojoules 1080, calories 258, protein 17.5g, fat 13g, saturated fat 3g, carbohydrate 15.5g, fibre 3.5g.

- Replace salmon with tuna for variety.
- Vita-Weat® or Ryvita® are suggested in this recipe as they are made from wholegrains. Other crackers can also be used, just look for wholemeal or wholegrain/multigrain varieties.

Tuna & Asparagus Crackers

Makes 4 cups

185g can tuna in spring water, drained and separated with a fork

1 spring onion, finely chopped

½ cup no added salt asparagus cuts and tips

Zest and juice of 1 lemon

1 red chilli, seeds removed and finely chopped

½ cup roughly chopped coriander (or parsley)

1 tomato, diced

8 Ryvita® crackers or 4 Vita-Weat® Lunch Slices

Combine the tuna, onion, asparagus, lemon zest and juice, chilli and coriander. Top with diced tomato. Spread evenly over crackers.

Nutrition information (per cup): kilojoules 585, calories 140, protein 12.5g, fat 3g, saturated fat 0.5, carbohydrate 13g, fibre 4.5g.

The toppings and fillings for crackers, pita bread and wraps can be swapped for different bases, as pictured.

Egg & Salad Wrap

Makes 4 cups

3 hard boiled eggs, chopped

½ cup corn kernels

1 tablespoon low fat mayonnaise

1 teaspoon curry powder (optional)

1 teaspoon white wine vinegar

1 tomato, chopped

Freshly ground black pepper

1-2 cups baby spinach, rocket or finely shredded lettuce

4 wholemeal mountain bread

Combine all ingredients except baby spinach and bread. Place filling to one side of the mountain bread. Top with baby spinach. Roll firmly to serve.

Nutrition information (per cup): kilojoules 695, calories 166, protein 9g, fat 5.5g, saturated fat 1.5g, carbohydrate 18.5g, fibre 3g.

- Some people with a gastric band find lettuce difficult to tolerate. You may find some varieties easier to tolerate than others, or you may prefer rocket or baby spinach. Experiment with different types and always shred the lettuce on your plate before eating.
- For perfect boiled eggs, place eggs in a saucepan and cover with cold water. Bring to the boil then gently boil, uncovered, stirring occasionally. Boil for 1 minute per egg for a soft boiled egg, 2 minutes per egg for a medium boiled egg and 3 minutes per egg for hard boiled eggs.

> "The Egg & Salad Wrap is suberb!"
> - Elaine, gastric band -

Beef & Mustard Pickle Wrap

Makes 4 cups

150g shaved roast beef, trimmed of fat, finely diced

¼ capsicum, finely diced

¼ cup sweet mustard pickle

¼ cup corn

1-2 cups baby spinach, rocket or finely shredded lettuce

4 wholemeal mountain bread

Combine beef, capsicum, corn and mustard pickle. Place filling to one side of each slice of mountain bread. Top with baby spinach. Roll firmly to serve.

Nutrition information (per cup): kilojoules 635, calories 152, protein 13g, fat 2.5g, saturated fat 1g, carbohydrate 17.5g, fibre 2.5g.

To avoid wraps, sandwiches or crackers going soggy in your lunchbox, combine fillings and take separately in a small plastic container. Assemble when you are ready to eat.

Chicken on Crackers

Makes 4 cups

150g cooked skinless chicken or turkey, shaved or diced

1 teaspoon dill, chopped

¼ cup low fat mayonnaise

½ cup cucumber, sliced or diced

½ avocado, diced

4 tablespoons cranberry sauce

8 Ryvita® crackers or 4 Vita-Weat® Lunch Slices

Combine chicken, dill, cucumber, avocado and mayonnaise. Spread crackers with cranberry sauce then top with chicken mixture.

Nutrition information (per cup): kilojoules 1160, calories 278, protein 13g, fat 14g, saturated fat 3g, carbohydrate 23.5g, fibre 3g.

Avocado on Crackers

Makes 4 cups

½ large avocado, skin removed, diced

½ teaspoon ground cumin

2 spring onions, finely diced

1 cup low fat cottage cheese

Juice of 1 lemon

1 tablespoon sweet chilli sauce

¼ cup fresh coriander, roughly chopped

8 Ryvita® crackers or 4 Vita-Weat® Lunch Slices

Combine avocado, cumin, spring onions, cottage cheese, lemon juice, sweet chilli sauce and coriander and mix well. Spread evenly on the crackers.

Nutrition information (per cup): kilojoules 840, calories 201, protein 13g, fat 8g, saturated fat 2g, carbohydrate 17g, fibre 3.5g.

If you would prefer this as a wrap, include shredded lettuce, baby spinach or rocket. Some grated carrot or diced cucumber may also be a nice addition.

"Really yummy. I used the regular Vitaweat® 9 Grain crackers and this was satisfying enough. You could possibly add a little tuna or chicken to the mixture, however it was very nice as it was....."
- *Leoni, gastric bypass -*

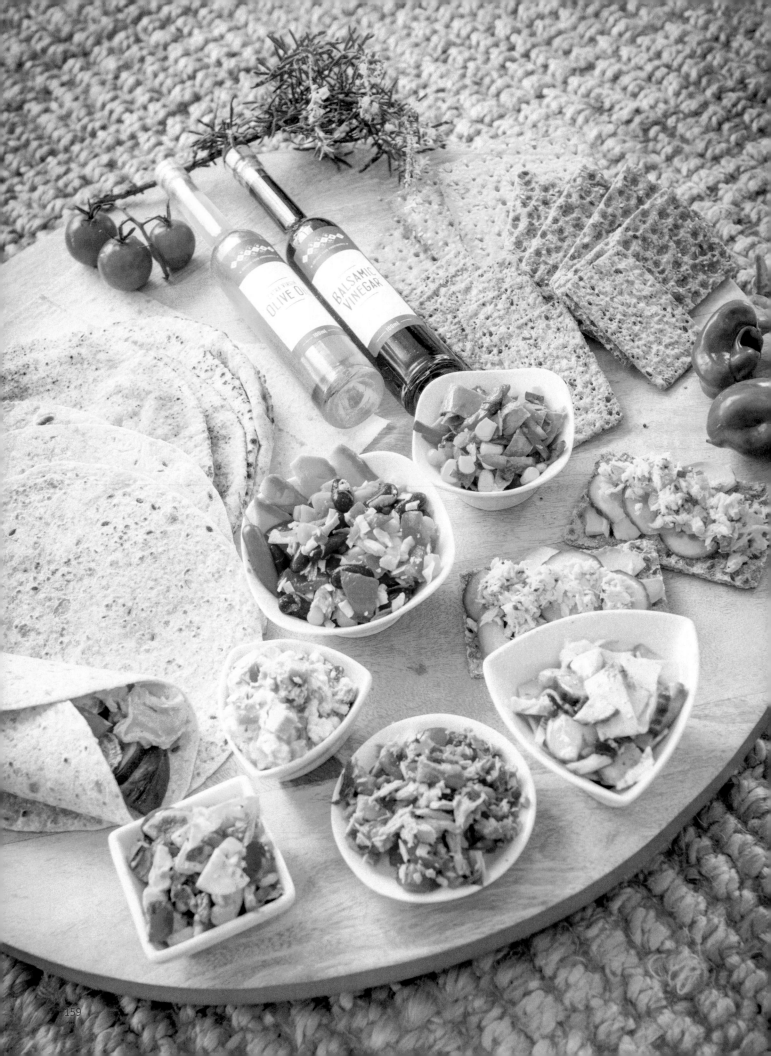

Dinner

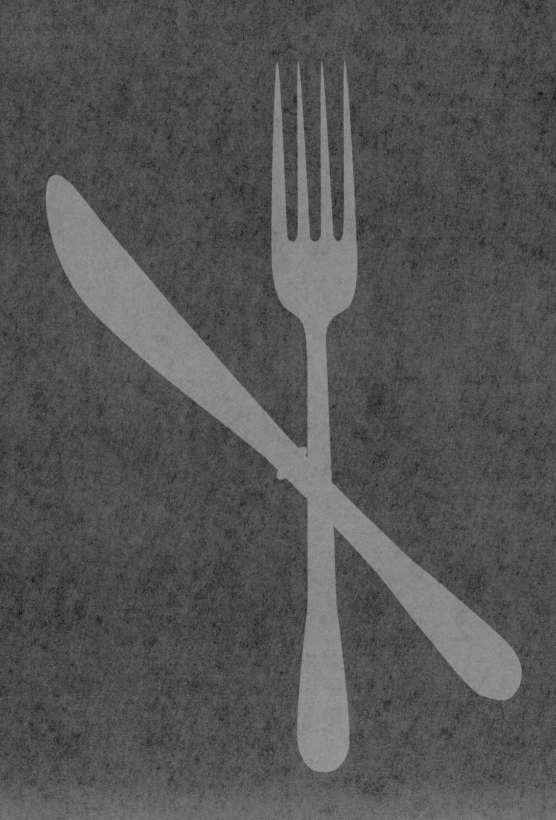

Oriental Beef

Makes 4 cups

400g beef, trimmed of fat, sliced thinly

1 tablespoon lime juice

1 tablespoon fresh ginger, grated

2 cloves garlic, crushed

1 tablespoon fresh basil leaves, finely shredded

1 tablespoon sesame oil

1 onion, sliced finely

¼ Chinese cabbage, finely shredded

1 bunch Bok Choy, or Choy Sum, finely shredded

2 tablespoons balsamic vinegar

Handful of snow peas (approximately 8), strings removed

Combine beef, lime juice, ginger, garlic, basil and 1 tablespoon of the balsamic vinegar. Cover and refrigerate for 3 hours or overnight. Drain beef and discard the marinade. Heat half of the sesame oil in a wok and stir-fry onion until soft. Add beef and stir-fry in batches until cooked as desired, then remove beef and set aside. Add cabbage, Bok Choy or Choy Sum, snow peas, remaining vinegar and oil to the wok. Stir-fry until the vegetables are just cooked. Return the beef to the wok. Toss until well combined and heated through.

Nutrition information (per cup): kilojoules 800, calories 191, protein 22.5g, fat 9.5g, saturated fat 2.5g, carbohydrate 2.5g, fibre 2g.

- If you have diabetes, include a smaller serve of stir-fry and a small amount of basmati rice or rice noodles.
- To help slice meat thinly, slice whilst partly frozen.

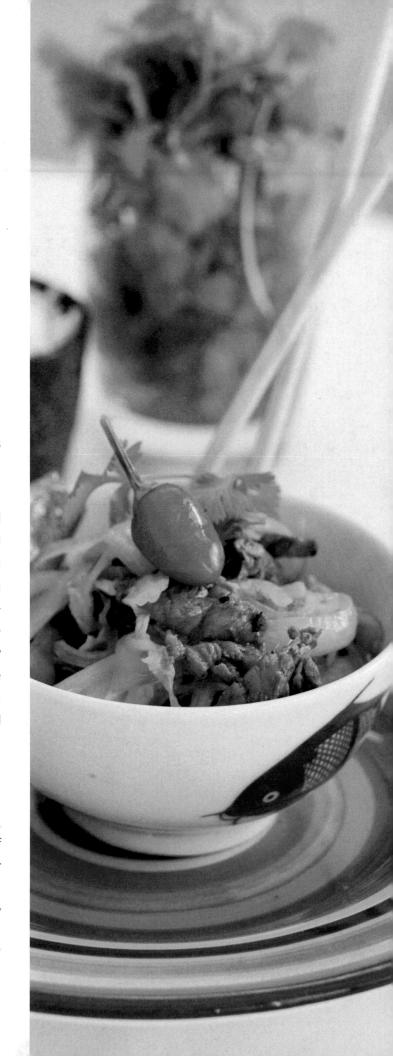

Chicken Stir-fry with Pine Nuts & Raisins

Makes 4 cups

1 tablespoon oil

400g skinless chicken, trimmed of fat, sliced thinly eg. breast, thigh or tenderloin

1 tablespoon lemon juice

2 teaspoons salt reduced soy sauce

1 teaspoon ginger, minced

2 cloves garlic, crushed

1 onion, quartered, separated into petals

1 red capsicum, cut into strips

1½ cups broccoli florets

2 tablespoons pine nuts

2 tablespoons raisins

Freshly ground black pepper

Combine chicken, lemon juice, soy and ginger in a bowl. Cover and refrigerate for 1-2 hours. Heat a saucepan with half of the oil. Stir-fry chicken over high heat, tossing until lightly browned. Remove chicken from pan and set aside. Heat the remaining oil in the saucepan. Add garlic and onion and cook over high heat, tossing, until the onion is cooked. Add the capsicum and broccoli and cook, stirring, until the vegetables are tender but still crisp. Add the pine nuts and raisins and cook for 2 minutes. Add chicken back to the pan and cook until heated through. Season with pepper to taste.

Nutrition information (per cup): kilojoules 1210, calories 289, protein 22.5g, fat 18g, saturated fat 3.5g, carbohydrate 8g, fibre 3g.

If you have diabetes, serve with a small serve of hokkien noodles. Larger appetites (family or friends) may also enjoy these as a side dish.

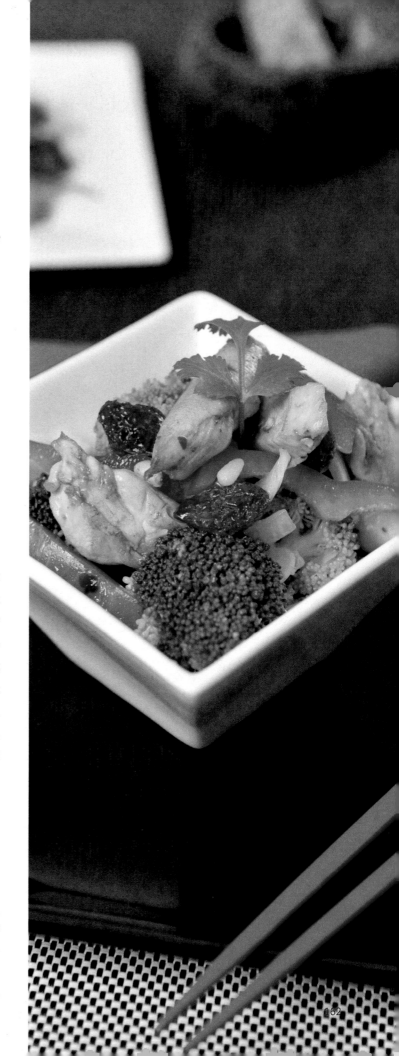

Mexican Fish Parcels with Spicy Mexican Salad

Makes 4 cups

4 x 125g fish fillets eg. salmon, barramundi

1 clove garlic, minced

1 teaspoon jalapeno peppers

Handful of fresh coriander, chopped

1 small green capsicum, half sliced and half diced

1 bunch spring onions, chopped

2 small tomatoes, 1 thinly sliced and 1 diced

½ cup red kidney beans

125g can corn kernels, drained

2 tablespoons pitted black olives, sliced

1 tablespoon chili sauce

1 teaspoon sugar

(or 1 tablespoon sweet chilli sauce instead of chili sauce and sugar)

1 tablespoon red wine vinegar

Dash of HP sauce

Nutrition information (per cup): kilojoules 910, calories 218, protein 29g, fat 3.5g, saturated fat 1g, carbohydrate 15g, fibre 4g.

Recipe inspiration courtesy of Sharon, gastric band.

Preheat oven to 180°C. Place 4 x 30cm squares of baking paper on top of 4 x 30cm squares of foil. Place fish fillet in centre of baking paper. Sprinkle each fillet with garlic and jalapenos. Top with fresh coriander, half of the sliced capsicum, half of the spring onions and sliced tomatoes. Fold into a parcel and bake for about 10-12 minutes then let stand for 5 minutes (fish will continue to cook from residual heat).

Whilst fish is cooking, combine the diced green capsicum, the diced tomato, half of the spring onions, kidney beans, corn and olives. Combine chilli sauce, sugar (or sweet chilli sauce), red wine vinegar, HP sauce in a small jar and shake well. Pour over salad to serve.

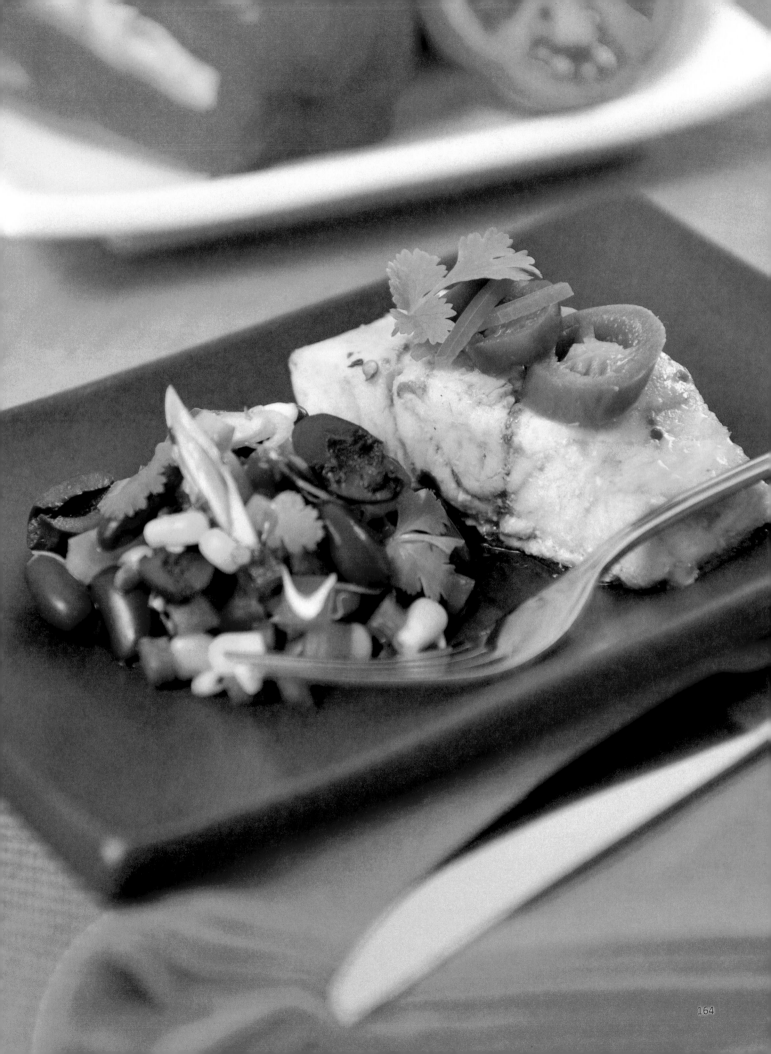

Fajitas

Makes 4 cups

Oil spray

400g beef, trimmed of fat, sliced thinly

¼ cup salt reduced barbeque sauce

1 teaspoon ground cumin

1 teaspoon ground coriander

½ teaspoon chilli powder

½ red onion, sliced

½ red capsicum, sliced

½ green capsicum, sliced

4 tortillas eg. Old El Paso®

4 teaspoons of extra light sour cream

Avocado Topping

½ avocado

1 teaspoon lime juice

½ clove garlic, crushed

Mash avocado with lime juice and garlic.

Tomato Salsa

1 tomato, seeded, diced

¼ red onion, diced

1 teaspoon fresh coriander, chopped

Combine all ingredients.

Combine beef in a bowl with sauce, cumin, coriander and chilli. Cover and refrigerate for 3 hours or overnight. Spray barbeque plate with oil BEFORE lighting barbeque. Cook onion, capsicum and beef on the barbeque until beef is cooked as

desired. Divide beef and vegetable mixture among 4 tortillas. Top each with Avocado Topping, Tomato Salsa and a teaspoon of sour cream.

Nutrition information (per cup): kilojoules 1345, calories 322, protein 25g, fat 15g, saturated fat 4.5g, carbohydrate 20.5g, fibre 2.5g.

For variety, use chicken in this recipe instead of beef.

"DELICIOUS!"
- Cathi, gastric band -

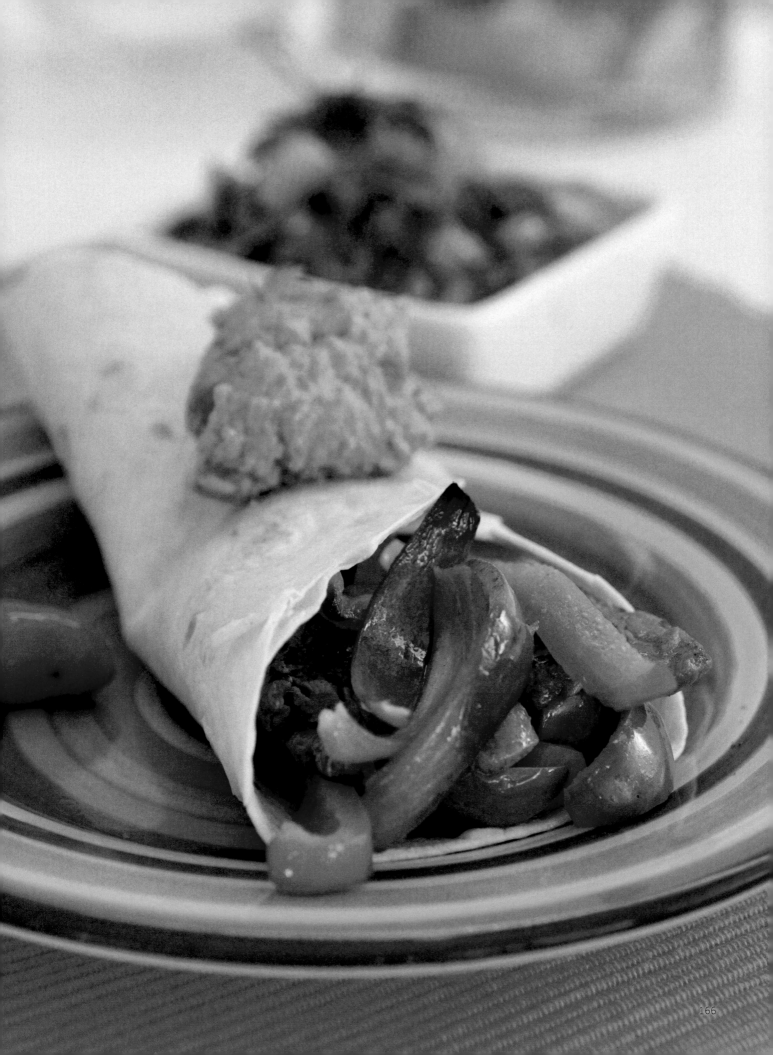

Pork Chow Mein

Makes 4 cups

2 teaspoons peanut oil

350g lean pork mince

2 garlic cloves, finely diced

3 spring onions, trimmed and thinly sliced diagonally

⅛ cabbage, finely shredded

½ red capsicum, thinly sliced

1 carrot, peeled into ribbons with a potato peeler

¼ cup frozen peas

½ cup water

1 teaspoons cornflour

2 tablespoons oyster sauce

1½ tablespoons soy sauce

100g Hokkien, thin egg or Singapore noodles

Cover noodles with boiling water and let stand for 1 minute or until tender. Drain noodles and separate with a fork. Set aside. Combine cornflour, water, oyster sauce and soy sauce in a jug and stir until smooth. Set aside. Heat the oil in a wok over high heat. Add the pork mince and garlic and stir-fry, breaking up the mince with a wooden as it is cooking. Cook for 3 to 4 minutes, or until the pork is cooked through. Add the onions, capsicum and carrots and stir-fry for 2 minutes. Add the sauce mixture and bring to the boil. Add the peas, cabbage and noodles and stir-fry for 2 to 3 minutes or until the peas are tender.

Nutrition information (per cup): kilojoules 760, calories182, protein 19.5g, fat 6.5g, saturated fat 2.5g, carbohydrate 10g, fibre 2.5g

This recipe is quite salty. If you have high blood pressure and need to limit salt, use this recipe occasionally only.

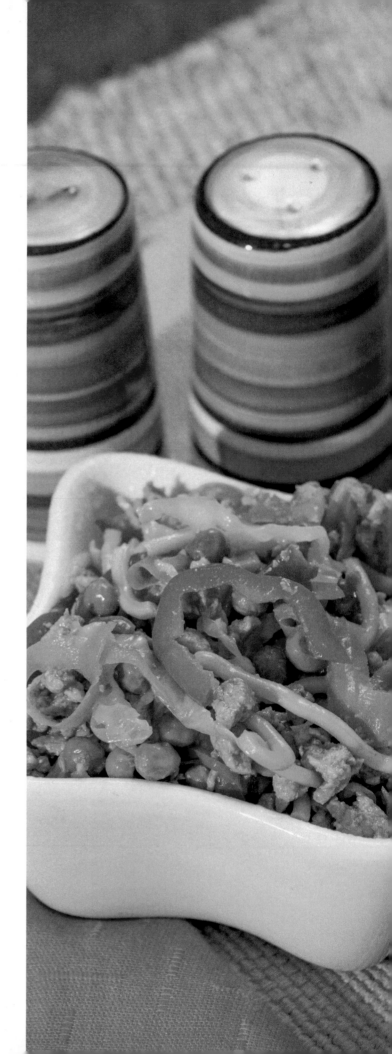

Chicken Kebabs

Makes 4 cups

500g skinless chicken eg. breast, thigh or tenderloin

½ red capsicum, cut into squares

½ zucchini, sliced

2 corn cobs, halved

Marinade

1 chilli, halved and seeded

½ onion, finely diced

2 teaspoons fresh ginger, grated

1 tablespoon lemon juice

2 tablespoons reduced salt soy sauce

2 teaspoons honey

2 teaspoons sesame or peanut oil

Cut chicken into 2cm cubes. Combine marinade ingredients in a jar and shake well. Pour over chicken, cover, refrigerate and marinate for 2 hours. Thread on to skewers, alternating chicken with pieces of zucchini and capsicum. Grill skewers and corn under a preheated grill or barbeque for 5-8 minutes, turning often, until chicken is browned. Serve chicken skewers with half a corn cob.

Nutrition information (per cup): kilojoules 1235, calories 295, protein 27.5g, fat 13g, saturated fat 3.5g, carbohydrate 14.5g, fibre 3g.

Use stainless steel skewers, or soak wooden skewers in water prior to use.

> **"I tried the chicken kebabs minus the chilli as I'm not a lover of spicy food. They were great."**
> - *Kerry, gastric bypass* -

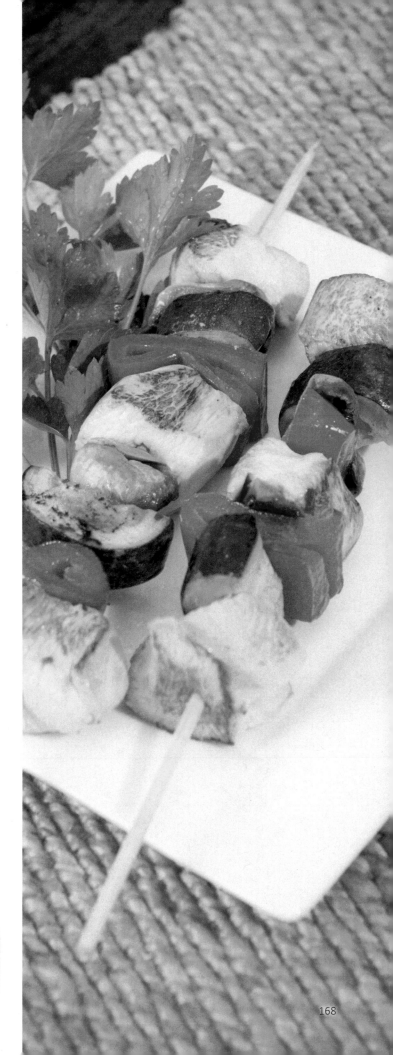

Chilli, Ginger & Lime Chicken

Makes 4 cups

1 tablespoon sesame oil

400g skinless chicken, trimmed of fat, sliced thinly eg. breast, tenderloin, thigh

1 cup water chestnuts

½ red capsicum, seeded and cut into thin strips

1 carrot, peeled and cut into strips

1 cup snow peas, strings removed and sliced

Marinade

2 teaspoons fresh ginger, grated

2 cloves garlic, crushed

1 tablespoon lemongrass, finely chopped

1 tablespoon soy or fish sauce

1 tablespoon chilli sauce

2 tablespoons lime juice

¼ cup loosely packed coriander leaves

Combine marinade ingredients in a jar and shake well. Pour over chicken, cover and refrigerate for 2 hours. Remove chicken from marinade. Heat sesame oil in frying pan. Stir-fry chicken, moving constantly, until lightly browned. Add water chestnuts, capsicum, carrot and snow peas. Stir-fry, moving constantly, until tender but still crisp.

Nutrition information (per cup): kilojoules 1010, calories 242, protein 21g, fat 13.5g, saturated fat 3.5g, carbohydrate 7.5g, fibre 3g.

- If you have diabetes, serve with a small amount of basmati rice or rice noodles. Larger appetites (family and friends) may also enjoy a serve of these.
- For variety, replace chicken with green prawn meat. Seafood does not need to marinate for as long as chicken - marinate for 10 - 20 minutes only. Follow the same method, however cook prawns and remove from pan before cooking vegetables. Return prawns once vegetables are cooked and heat through.

"We love Asian flavours and this recipe is simply delicious. My children have requested this dish time and time again."
- Robyn, gastric bypass -

"I really loved the flavours in this recipe - sweet and tangy. It was quite filling and the recipe was very easy to follow."
- Leoni, gastric bypass -

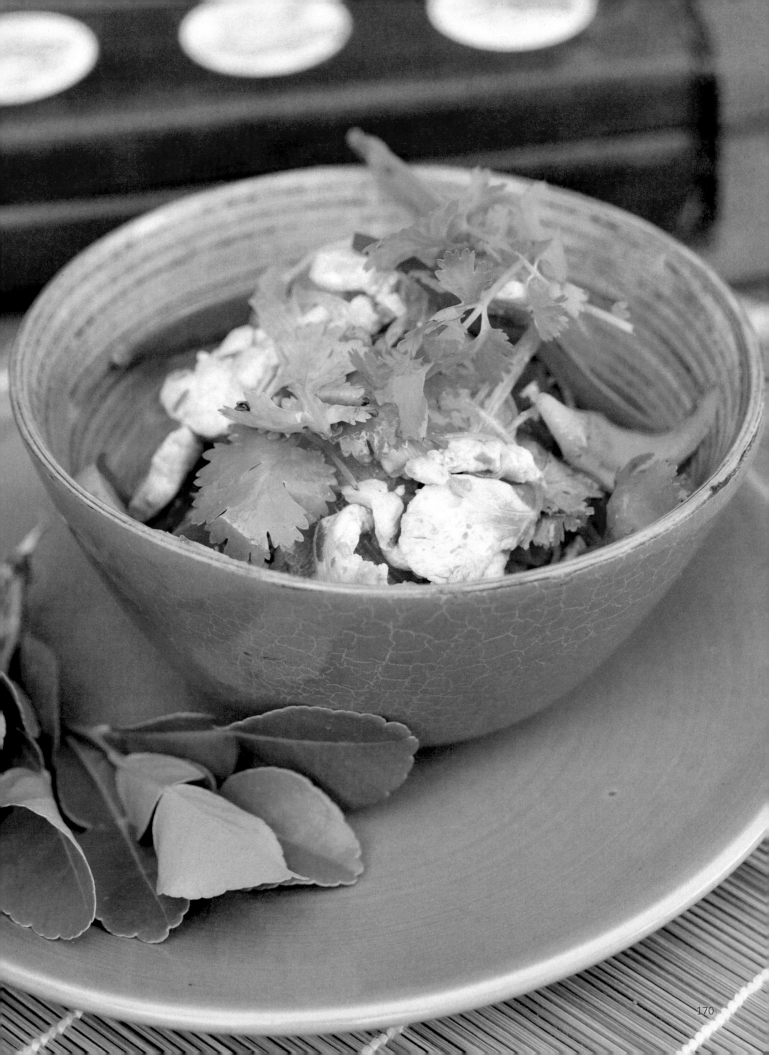

Zesty Tomato Fish S*

Makes 4 cups

Oil spray

500g firm white fish fillets

2 tablespoons salt reduced soy sauce

1 tablespoon salt reduced tomato sauce

1 tablespoon lemon juice

Vegetable kebabs

1 small zucchini, cut into 2cm chunks

1 red capsicum, cut into 2cm chunks

1 cup mushrooms, stalk removed, brushed clean and halved

1 cup cherry tomatoes

1 tablespoon salt reduced soy sauce

1 clove garlic, crushed

- Use stainless steel skewers or soak wooden skewers in water prior to use to prevent burning.
- S* This recipe is suitable on the soft diet if you ensure the vegetable kebabs are cooked until tender so the vegetables can be broken with the side of a fork.

Combine soy sauce, tomato sauce and lemon juice and pour over fish in a shallow dish. Cover with and marinate for 1 hour. To make kebabs, place all ingredients in a small plastic bag and seal. Shake and rub ingredients together until well combined. Thread vegetables onto skewers and place on a preheated barbeque or non-stick frying pan that has been sprayed with oil. Cook 15-20 minutes until vegetables are tender. Remove fish from marinade, reserving marinade and add to a preheated barbeque or frying pan. Cook fish for a few minutes each side, until fish is tender, brushing with the reserved marinade during cooking. Serve fish with vegetable kebabs.

Nutrition information (per cup): kilojoules 720, calories 172, protein 28g, fat 4g, saturated fat 1g, carbohydrate 4g, fibre 2g.

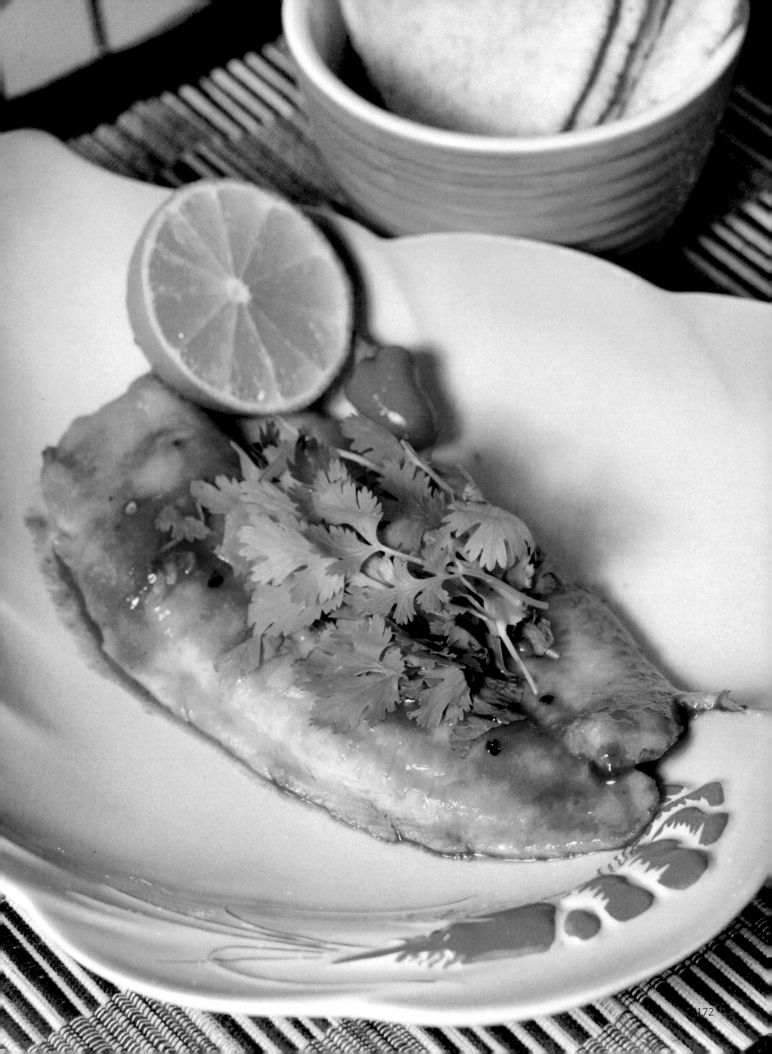

Lamb & Rosemary Kebabs

Makes 4 cups

500g lamb, trimmed of fat, cubed

2 teaspoons olive oil

½ tablespoon fresh rosemary

1 potato, peeled, cut into chunks

1 carrot, peeled, cut into chunks

1 onion, cut into chunks

½ cup peas (frozen)

Marinade

2 teaspoons olive oil

½ cup dry red wine

1 tablespoon salt reduced soy sauce

1 clove garlic, crushed

½ - 1 tablespoon fresh rosemary, chopped

½ red onion, finely chopped

Freshly ground black pepper

- Use stainless steel skewers, or soak wooden skewers in water prior to use to avoid scorching.
- If you have diabetes, add some sweet potato to the vegetables as a side dish.

Place lamb in a large shallow dish. Combine marinade ingredients, pour over lamb and mix well so lamb is well coated. Cover and refrigerate 3 hours or overnight. Preheat oven to 180°C. Combine vegetables, oil and rosemary in a bag or bowl and mix well to coat. Bake vegetables in the oven for 20 minutes or until cooked. Preheat barbeque. Drain lamb and discard marinade. Thread lamb on skewers and cook on a barbeque until browned all over and cooked as desired. Steam peas and serve lamb with vegetables.

Nutrition information (per cup): kilojoules 1150, calories 275, protein 28.5g, fat 13.5g, saturated fat 4.5g, carbohydrate 7g, fibre 2.5g.

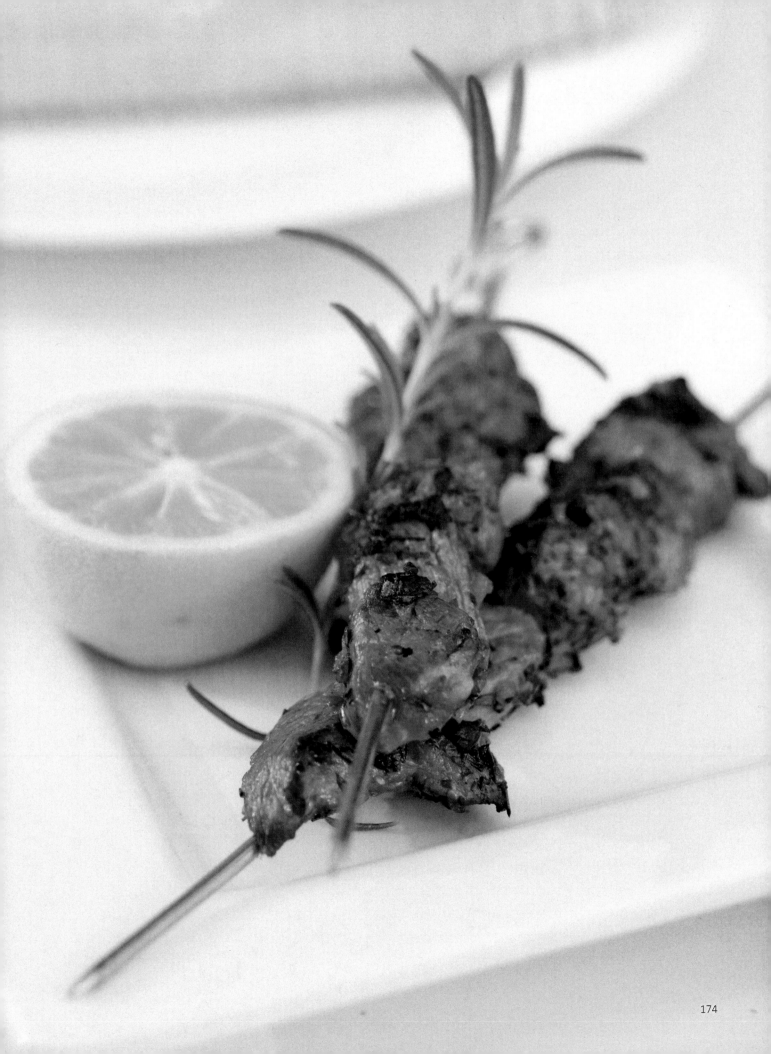

Prawn Paella

Makes 4 cups

Oil spray

1 red onion, sliced

3 cloves of garlic, crushed

½ chorizo sausage

2 teaspoons sweet paprika

¼ cup Arborio rice

½ red capsicum, chopped

1 cup no added salt, chopped tinned tomatoes

¾ cup salt reduced chicken stock

A pinch of saffron threads, soaked in 1 tablespoon hot water

Chilli flakes, to taste

300g green prawns

⅓ cup of frozen peas

⅓ cup flat leaf parsley, roughly chopped, to serve

4 lemon wedges, to serve

Nutrition information (per cup): kilojoules 785, calories 188, protein 20g, fat 4.5g, saturated fat 1g, carbohydrate 15.5g, fibre 2.5g.

Recipe inspiration courtesy of Sharon, gastric band.

Peel the papery skin off of the chorizo sausage, slice thinly and cut each slice in half. Heat a non sitck frying pan that has been sprayed with oil. Add onion, garlic and sausage and cook over a medium heat for 3 minutes, or until onion has softened. Add paprika and rice and cook for a minute until the rice is well coated. Add capsicum and cook for 1-2 minutes. Pour in the tomatoes, stock and saffron. Sprinkle with chilli if desired. Stir and bring to the boil. Reduce heat and simmer gently for 15 minutes, stirring occasionally. (The rice may stick to the bottom of the pan - this is normal in paella, but just give it a stir to move it.) Add the prawns and peas to the paella stir and cook for a further 3 minutes or until the prawns are cooked and rice is tender. Serve sprinkled with parsley and a lemon wedge.

"Tasty and satisfying!"
- Sharon, gastric band -

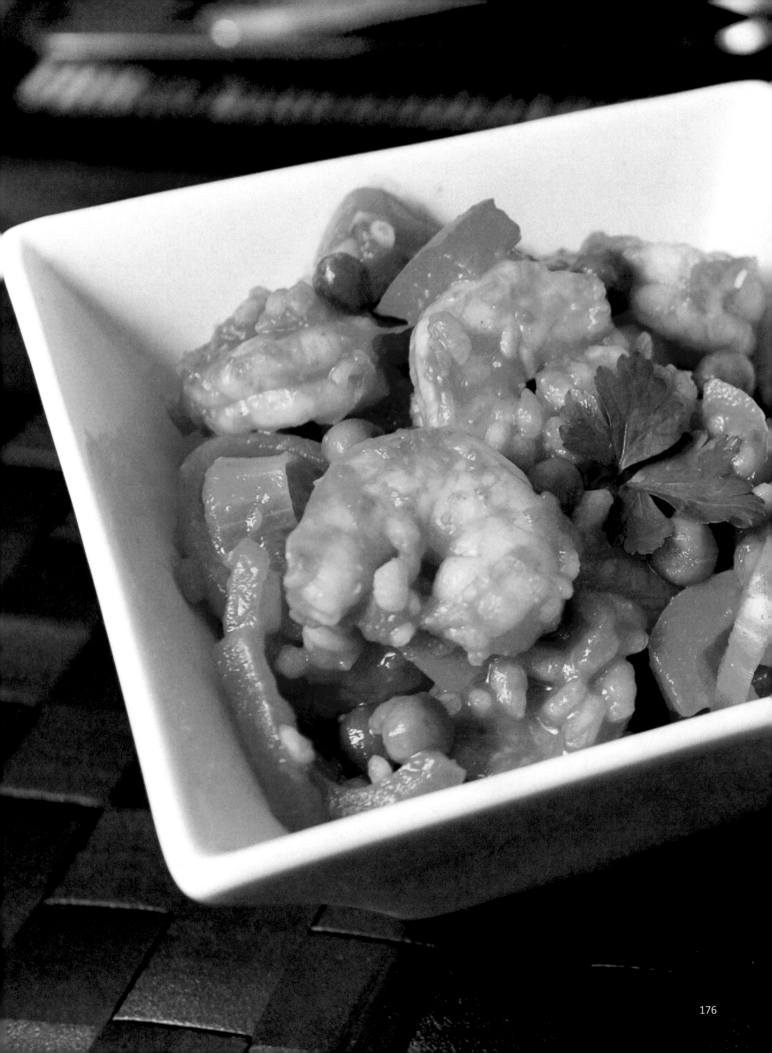

Baked Salmon & Cauliflower Puree

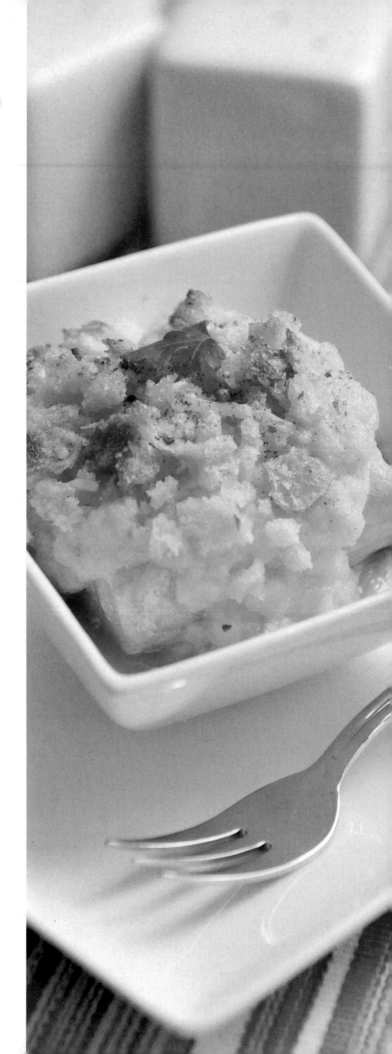

Makes 4 cups

500g salmon (4 x 125g pieces), skin removed

½ onion, chopped

1-2 cloves garlic, crushed

2 cups cauliflower florets

½ parsnip, peeled and chopped

¼ cup cannellini beans, drained and rinsed

1 teaspoon vegetable stock powder

¾ cup low fat milk

1 tablespoon dried bread crumbs

Pre-heat oven to 200°C. Combine onion, garlic, cauliflower, parsnip, vegetable stock powder and milk in a large saucepan. (Use a large or deep saucepan because the milk can overflow when it is brought to the boil.) Place over medium heat and bring to the boil. As soon as it boils reduce the heat to low and let gently simmer until the vegetables are tender. Add the beans and remove from heat. Let cool for a few minutes.

Meanwhile, heat a non-stick frying pan that has been sprayed with a little oil over a medium to hot heat. Add the salmon and brown on each side for about 1 minute. Then place into a small baking dish. Puree the cauliflower mixture until smooth and pour over the fish. Sprinkle with breadcrumbs and bake in the oven for 15-20 minutes or until the fish cooked to your liking.

Nutrition information (per cup): kilojoules 1040, calories 249, protein 29.5g, fat 9.5g, saturated fat 2g, carbohydrate 10g, fibre 2.5g.

Recipe inspiration courtesy of Sharon, gastric band.

Bean & Vegetable Hot Pot S*

Makes 4 cups

Oil spray

1 onion, diced

1 tablespoon salt reduced soy sauce or Worcestershire sauce

1 clove garlic, crushed

1 cup salt reduced vegetable stock

1 carrot, diced

½ cup sweet potato, diced

½ zucchini, diced

½ red capsicum, diced

1⅓ cups cooked kidney beans (or 400g can kidney beans, drained and rinsed)

1 cup no added salt, tomato pasta sauce

1 teaspoon curry powder

3 tablespoons (45g) whey protein isolate powder

Heat a frying pan that has been sprayed with oil. Add onion, carrot, sweet potato and garlic, stirring until vegetables are tender. Add zucchini, capsicum, curry powder, soy sauce and stock, keeping 1/4 cup stock in reserve. Bring to the boil and simmer for 2-3 minutes. Add kidney beans and pasta sauce and simmer for 5-10 minutes. Dissolve protein powder in the reserved stock and stir through.

Nutrition information (per cup): kilojoules 730, calories 175, protein 17g, fat 2.5g, saturated fat 0.5g, carbohydrate 18.5g, fibre 7g.

- Larger appetites (family and friends) may enjoy pasta or cous cous as a side dish.
- Suitable to freeze.
- **S*** This recipe is suitable on the soft diet if you ensure the vegetables are cooked until tender and can be broken with the side of a fork.

> "I really like this recipe.
> I have passed it on to friends who also enjoyed it."
> - *Pam, gastric band -*

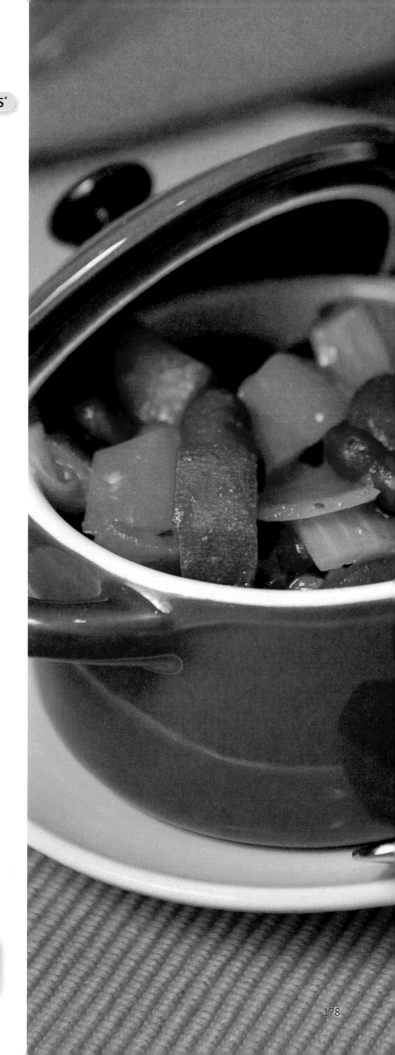

Spicy Barbeque Fish Wraps

Makes 4 cups

500g firm white fish fillets

4 tablespoons lemon juice

1 teaspoon freshly ground pepper

2 teaspoons ground turmeric

1 onion, finely grated

2 cloves garlic, crushed

2 teaspoons fresh ginger, grated

2 teaspoons ground coriander

2 teaspoons ground cumin

¼ teaspoon ground cinnamon

1 teaspoon lemon zest

½ teaspoon chilli powder

Lettuce, finely shredded, to serve

Tomato, sliced, to serve

Cucumber, sliced, to serve

4 slices wholemeal mountain bread

Slash fish a couple of times on each side. Combine lemon juice, grated onion and herbs. Mix to a paste and spread all over the fish. Wrap each fish in foil. Place on preheated barbeque (or under a preheated grill) for 7-10 minutes on each side or until fish flakes when tested with a fork. Open foil for the last few minutes to allow excess moisture to evaporate. Divide fish between mountain bread. Top with salad and wrap firmly to serve.

Nutrition information (per cup): kilojoules 940, calories 225, protein 29.5g, fat 3.5g, saturated fat 1g, carbohydrate 16.5g, fibre 3g.

For variety, stuff fish and salad into a small wholemeal pita pocket instead of serving as a wrap.

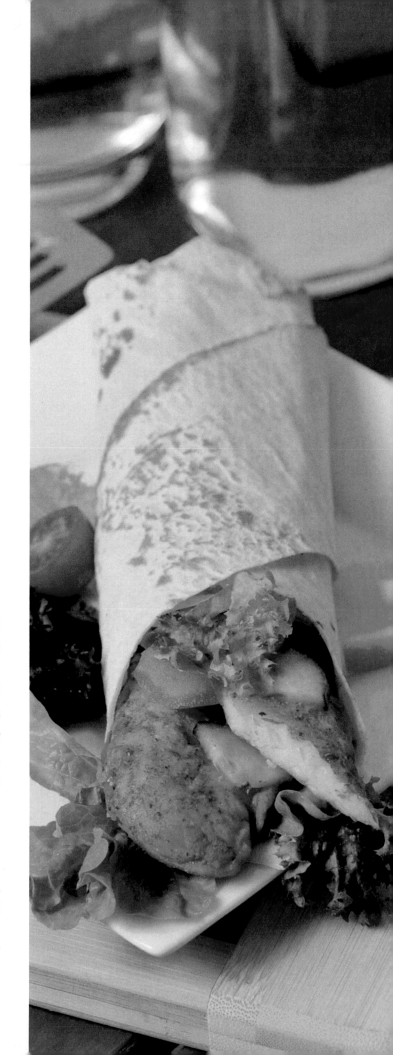

Stuffed Capsicums S*

Makes 4 cups

Oil spray

1 onion, finely diced

2 cloves garlic, crushed

400g lean mince eg. premium or extra trim

1 large tomato, diced

1 tablespoon no added salt tomato paste

Freshly ground black pepper

2 tablespoons parsley, chopped

4 small-medium capsicums, or 2 large capsicums

1 cup no added salt tomato pasta sauce

Preheat oven to 200°C. Cut tops from small-medium capsicums or halve large capsicums lengthways. Scrape out seeds and pith. (If you have used small-medium capsicums, set aside the tops and dice.) Heat a frying pan that has been sprayed with oil. Add onions and garlic (and diced capsicum if reserved) and cook gently until softened. Add the mince and stir well, breaking up lumps, until browned. Stir in tomato, tomato paste, ½ cup tomato pasta sauce, pepper and parsley. Simmer for another minute or two until the liquid has reduced. Fill each capsicum with some of the meat mixture and stand in a baking dish that has been sprayed with oil. Add a dollop of the remaining pasta sauce to the capsicums before baking. Cover dish with a lid or foil and cook in the oven for about 40 minutes.

Nutrition information (per cup): kilojoules 1050, calories 251, protein 25g, fat 9g, saturated fat 3g, carbohydrate 14.5g, fibre 5.5g.

- Larger appetites (family and friends) may enjoy a simple green side salad.
- The mince filling can be frozen to use later.
- S* The mince filling is suitable on the soft diet.

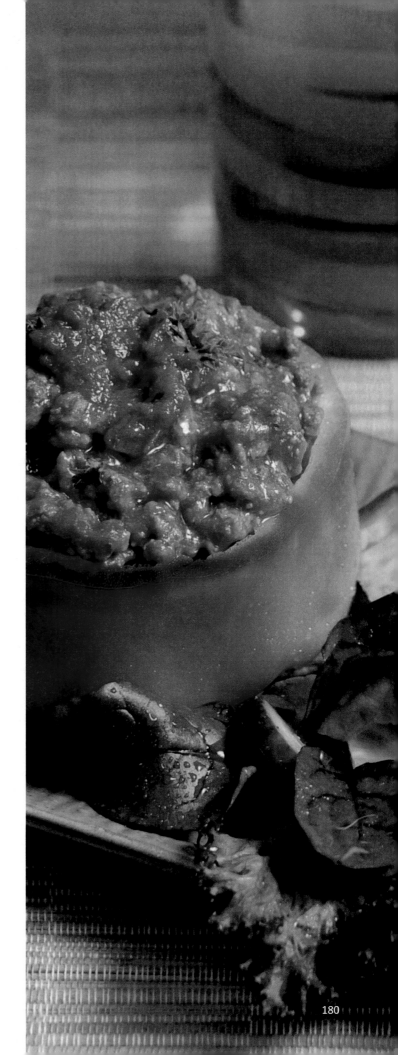

Meatballs with Vegetable Sauce S

Makes 4 cups

Meatballs

Oil spray

400g lean mince eg. premium/extra trim

½ onion, grated

2 tablespoons sultanas, chopped

¼ cup fresh parsley, chopped

1 tablespoon no added salt tomato paste

1 tablespoon wholemeal plain flour

Freshly ground black pepper

Combine mince, onion, sultanas, parsley, pepper and tomato paste. Mix well and shape into 20 small balls. Spread flour over a clean bench or baking paper. Roll meatballs in flour to lightly coat. Heat a frying pan sprayed with oil. Add meatballs and brown all over.

Vegetable Sauce

1 clove garlic, crushed

2 tablespoons no added salt tomato paste

½ cup dry red wine

½ cup salt reduced beef stock

½ cup no added salt, chopped tinned tomatoes

1 bay leaf

½ teaspoon dried oregano (optional)

½ teaspoon dried thyme (optional)

½ teaspoon basil (optional)

½ cup zucchini, diced

½ cup carrots, finely diced

5 mushrooms, quartered

½ cup cooked cannelini beans

Combine garlic, tomato paste, wine, stock, tinned tomatoes, bay leaf, oregano, thyme and basil, pour over meatballs. Add vegetables and beans and stir. Heat to boiling, lower heat and cook gently for 30-40 minutes or until vegetables are tender. Serve meatballs with vegetable sauce.

Nutrition information (per cup): kilojoules 1055, calories 252, protein 24.5g, fat 8.5g, saturated fat 3g, carbohydrate 15g, fibre 5g.

Larger appetites (family and friends) may enjoy oven baked potatoes topped with a spoonful of low fat natural yoghurt, or pasta as a side dish.

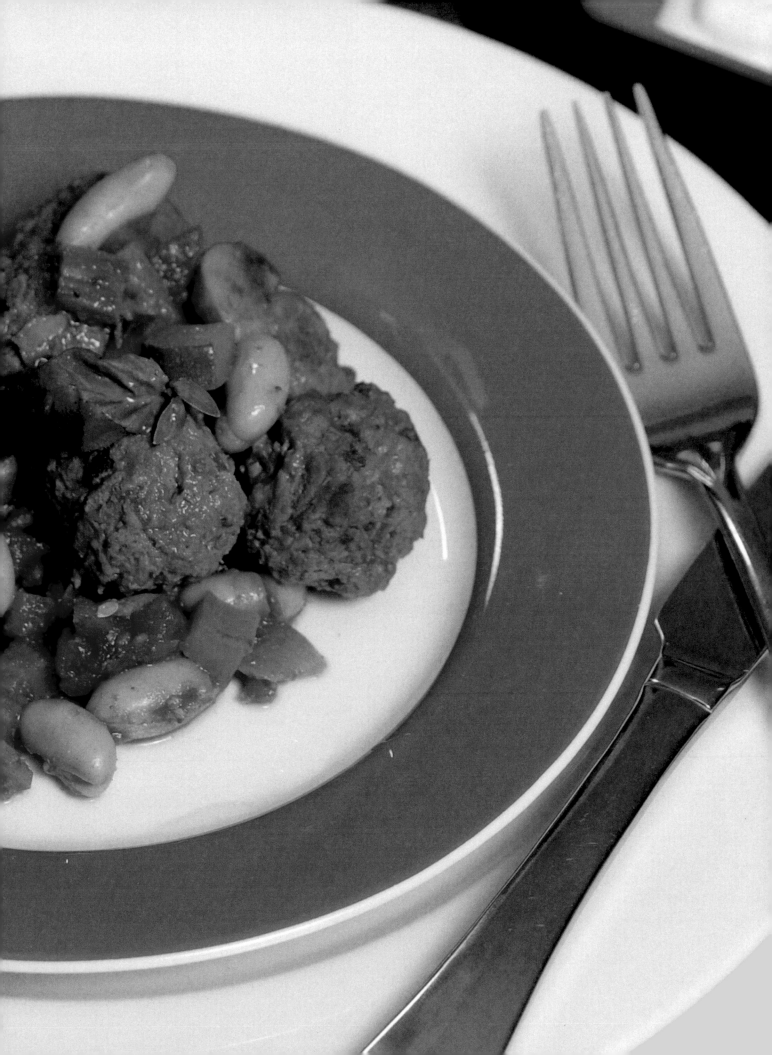

Vietnamese Beef & Mint Salad

Makes 4 cups

Oil spray

300g lean beef eg. Sirloin

½ cup mint leaves, shredded

1 cup savoy cabbage, shredded very finely

½ cup bean sprouts

1 small carrot, peeled into thin ribbons with a potato peeler

1 tablespoon crushed peanuts, toasted

Marinade/Dressing

1 tablespoon fish sauce

2 tablespoons water

1 teaspoon of sugar

2 tablespoons lime juice

1 clove garlic, crushed

½ teaspoon chilli powder

Combine ingredients for marinade/dressing in a jar and shake well to combine. Slice steak into thin strips and place in a bowl with half the mint leaves and marinade/dressing. Leave to marinate for about 30 minutes. Combine cabbage, bean sprouts, carrot, peanuts and remaining mint leaves in a bowl. Heat a frying pan or barbeque that has been sprayed with oil. Drain beef well, then add to the pan or barbeque and cook, stirring, until just cooked. Thin strips will cook quickly; take care not to overcook or beef will become tough. Combine beef, salad and dressing to serve.

Nutrition information (per cup): kilojoules 615, calories 146, protein 18g, fat 6g, saturated fat 2g, carbohydrate 3.5g, fibre 2.5g.

If you have diabetes, add some cooked Basmati rice or rice noodles to the salad to serve.

Recipe suggestion courtesy of Mercy Bariatrics.

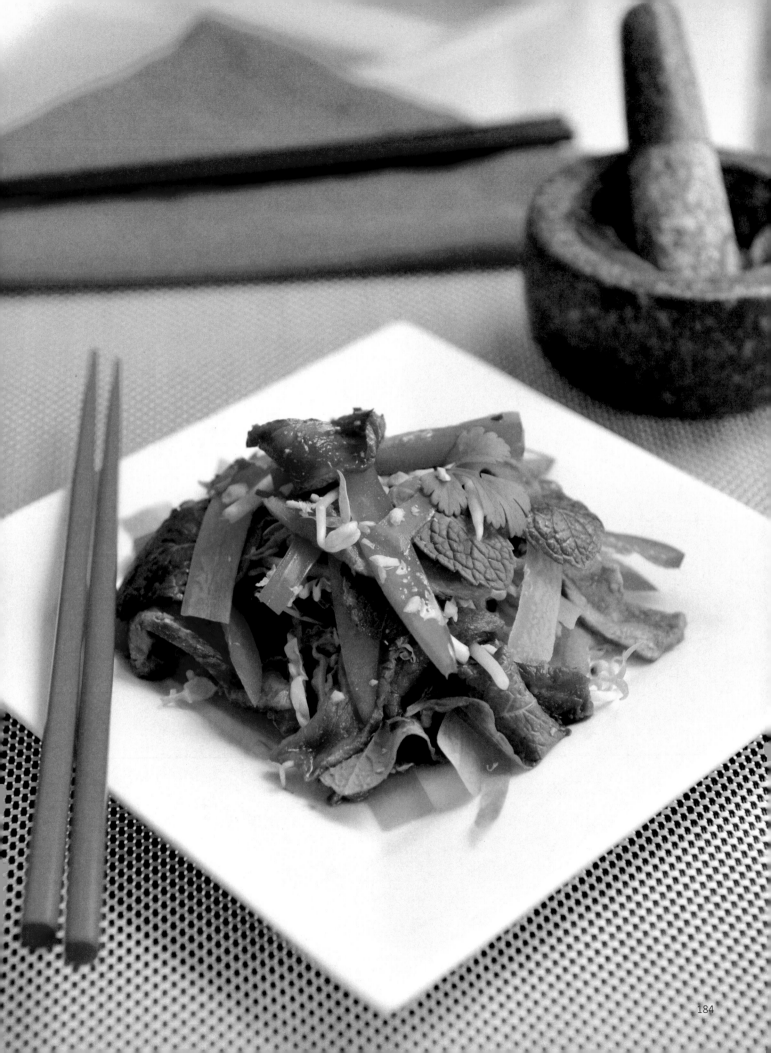

Middle Eastern Lamb S

Makes 4 cups

2 teaspoons oil

1 onion, sliced

1 teaspoon ground cinnamon

1 teaspoon ground cumin

400g lamb, trimmed of fat, diced

2 tablespoons fresh mint, chopped

1 tablespoon lemon rind, finely grated

1 cup salt reduced beef stock

400g no added salt, chopped tinned tomatoes

1 tablespoon honey

1⅓ cups cooked chickpeas (or 400g can chickpeas, drained and rinsed)

Heat oil in wok over medium heat. Add onion, cinnamon and cumin. Stir-fry approximately 3 minutes or until the onion is soft. Add lamb and stir-fry for 5 minutes or until brown. Add mint, lemon, rind, stock, tomatoes and honey to wok. Reduce heat, cover and simmer 40 minutes. Add chickpeas half way through cooking. Simmer until lamb is tender.

Nutrition information (per cup): kilojoules 1175, calories 281, protein 25.5g, fat 10.5g, saturated fat 3.5g, carbohydrate 18.5g, fibre 4.5g.

Suitable to freeze.

> **"The smells in the kitchen were amazing when I made this last night."**
>
> *- Russell, gastric band -*

> **"Wow!!!! 12 out of 10 from my wife and myself. The aromatics and flavours from the blending of cinnamon, cumin and mint were just amazing."**
>
> *- David, gastric band -*

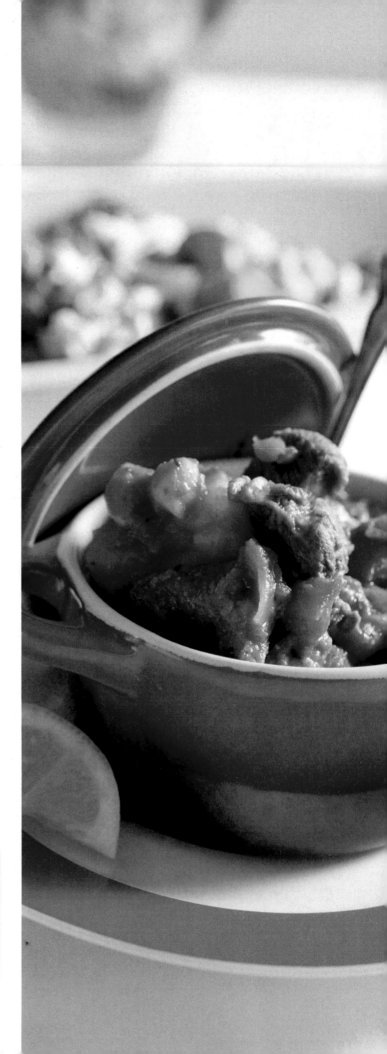

Beef in Red Wine

Makes 4 cups

1 tablespoon olive oil

500g beef steak, trimmed of fat

½ cup red wine

½ onion, sliced

1 bay leaf, crumbled

4 stalks parsley, chopped

½ teaspoon dried tarragon, thyme or oregano

Freshly ground black pepper

Place beef in a glass or ceramic dish. Mix remaining ingredients and pour over steak. Cover and leave to marinate in refrigerator for several hours, turning occasionally. Remove steak and place under a preheated grill or barbeque. Cook for approximately 3 minutes each side until sealed, then reduce heat and cook until desired tenderness. Baste with marinade during cooking and turn steak with tongs so that juices will not escape. Serve with Baby Spinach with Lemon (page 40).

Nutrition information (per cup): kilojoules 1000, calories 239, protein 29g, fat 10.5g, saturated fat 3g, carbohydrate 3g, fibre 2.5g.

- If you have diabetes, serve with a small serve of corn, potato, or oven baked sweet potato. Larger appetites (family and friends) may also enjoy these.
- If you don't have any red wine, use balsamic vinegar.

> "I thoroughly enjoyed this meal and all its flavours."
> *- Bec, gastric band -*

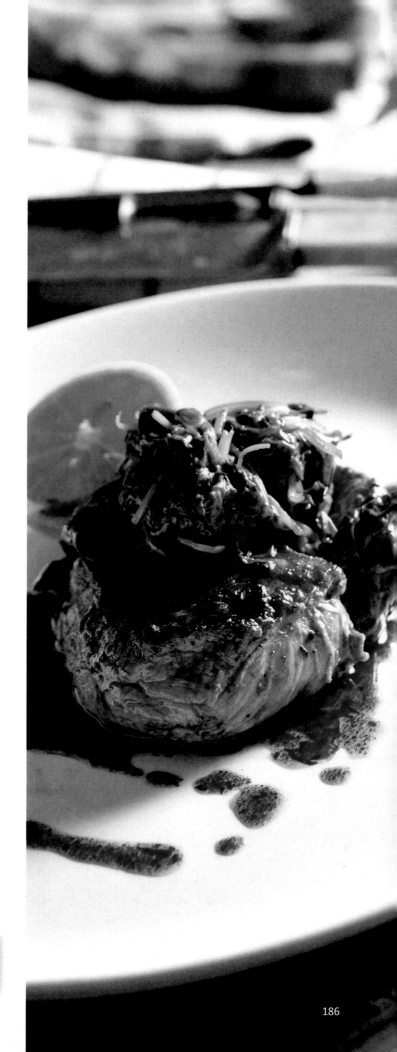

Creamy Vegetable Curry S*

Makes 4 cups

Oil spray

1 onion, chopped

2 cloves garlic, crushed

1 tablespoon diced fresh chilli or 2 teaspoons sliced dried chillies

1 teaspoon ground cumin

1 teaspoon cardamom

½ teaspoon garam marsala

2 teaspoons ground coriander

1 teaspoon ginger, grated

½ teaspoon ground turmeric

1⅓ cups cooked chickpeas (or 400g can chickpeas, drained and rinsed)

½ cup vegetable stock

1 cup sweet potato, peeled and diced

1 tomato, cut into wedges

½ cup green beans, trimmed and sliced

1 capsicum, seeded and sliced

½ cup low fat evaporated milk

1/4 cup water

2 tablespoons (30g) whey protein isolate powder

Freshly ground black pepper

Heat a wok or frying pan that has been sprayed with oil. Add the onion and stir-fry for 1-2 minutes. Add the garlic and spices. Cook gently for 2 minutes, stirring all the time. Add the chickpeas and stock and stir the mixture until it comes to the boil. Add the sweet potato, tomato, green beans and capsicum. Cover and cook over medium heat for approximately 15 minutes or until the sweet potato is tender. Dissolve protein powder in water and combine with evaporated milk. Stir through until well combined. Season to taste with pepper.

Nutrition information (per cup): kilojoules 765, calories 183, protein 15g, fat 3.5g, saturated fat 1g, carbohydrate 20.5g, fibre 5g.

- Larger appetites (family or friends) may enjoy basmati rice or cous cous as a side dish.
- To save time, replace the spices in this recipe with 2 tablespoons commercial Indian curry paste eg. Tikka Marsala.
- Suitable to freeze.
- S* This recipe is suitable on the soft diet if you ensure the vegetables are cooked until tender and can be broken with the side of a fork.

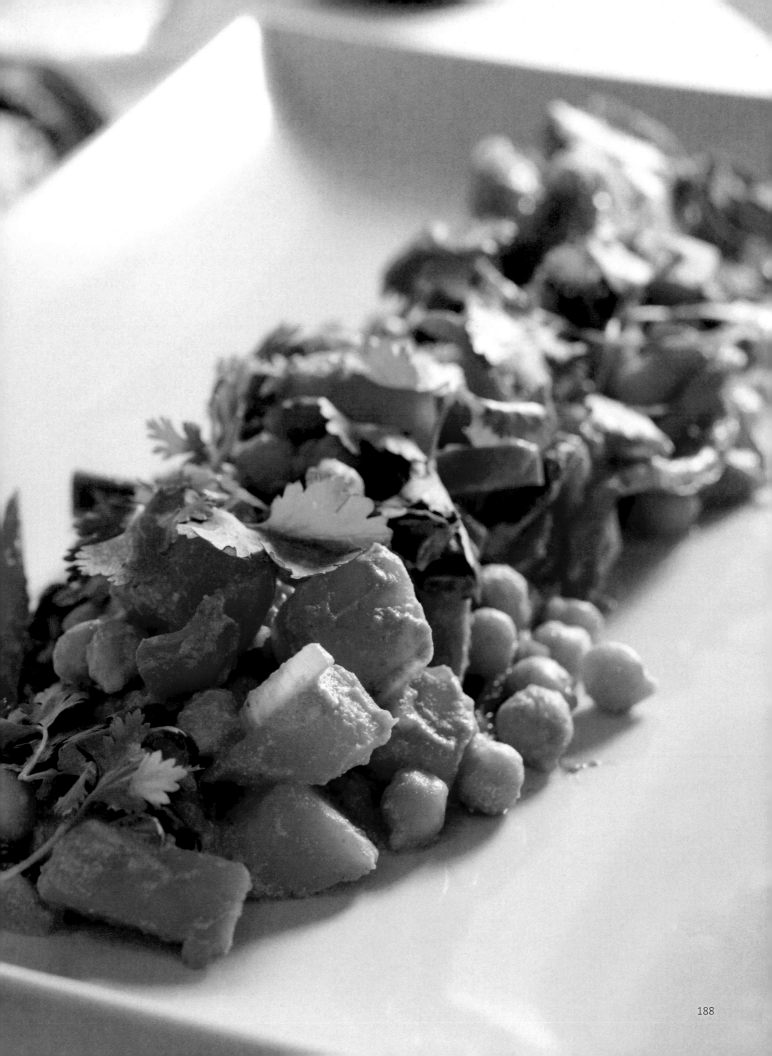

Tasty Tomato Beef S*

Makes 4 cups

Oil spray

500g beef, trimmed of fat, diced

1 clove garlic

1 onion, diced

2 tablespoons vinegar

1 packet salt reduced tomato soup mix

400g no added salt, chopped tinned tomatoes

1 tablespoon brown sugar

2 tablespoons sultanas

1 bay leaf

1 carrot, diced

½ cup green beans, sliced

Place all ingredients, except vegetables in a slow cooker and cook for approximately 9 hours. Add vegetables 2-3 hours before serving or once the beef is ready to serve, steam the vegetables and serve on the side. Stir occasionally. Serve with steamed cauliflower.

Nutrition information (per cup): kilojoules 1090, calories 261, protein 28.5g, fat 7.5g, saturated fat 3g, carbohydrate 18g, fibre 3g.

- If you don't have a slow cooker, brown beef in a large saucepan that has been sprayed with oil. Add the remaining ingredients (except vegetables) and bring to the boil. Reduce heat to very low and let simmer very gently for 2-3 hours. Add water as required to ensure the mixture is moist. Add the vegetables in the last hour.
- Family or friends may like plain or sweet potato mashed with low fat milk or a small baked potato with this dish.
- Suitable to freeze.
- **S*** This recipe is suitable on the soft diet if you ensure the vegetables are cooked until tender and can be broken with the side of a fork.

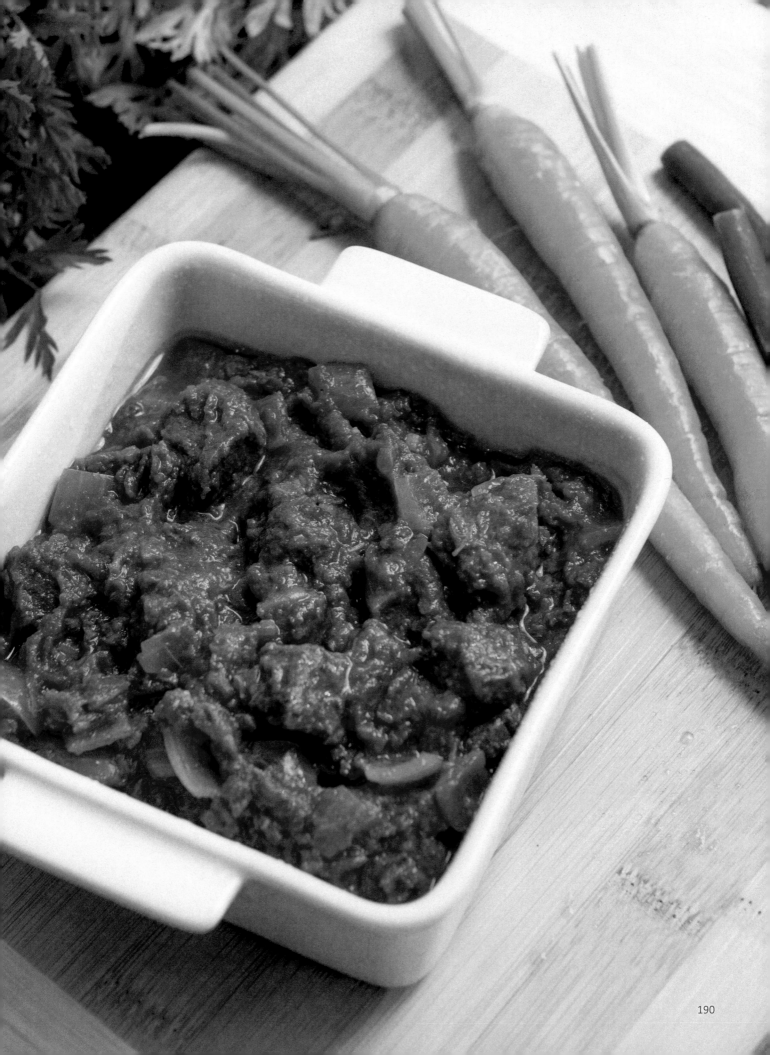

Chicken Creole S*

Makes 4 cups

2 teaspoons oil

500g skinless chicken, trimmed of fat, diced eg. thigh, breast or tenderloin

1 tablespoon wholemeal plain flour

1 onion, sliced

1 clove garlic, minced

1 green capsicum, chopped

1 stalk celery, chopped

2 teaspoons brown sugar

400g no added salt, chopped tinned tomatoes

2 teaspoons thyme

1 teaspoon basil

1 teaspoon Cajun seasoning

1 bay leaf, crumbled

Dash of Tabasco sauce

Freshly ground black pepper

½ lemon, sliced

1 tablespoon parsley, chopped

1 spring onion, sliced

Spread flour on a clean bench or baking paper. Roll diced chicken in flour. Heat a frying pan that has been sprayed with oil. Add chicken to pan and brown lightly. Remove chicken. Add onion, garlic, capsicum and celery. Gently cook for approximately 5 minutes. Add tinned tomatoes, sugar, thyme, basil, Cajun seasoning, bay leaf, Tabasco and pepper. Bring to the boil, then add chicken. Cover tightly, and simmer 40 minutes. In the last 15 minutes of cooking add lemon slices. Stir through parsley and spring onion just before serving.

Nutrition information (per cup): kilojoules 1095, calories 262, protein 26g, fat 13g, saturated fat 3.5g, carbohydrate 9g, fibre 2.5g.

- Larger appetites (family and friends) may enjoy a side serve of pasta.
- After gastric band surgery, some people find chicken breast difficult to tolerate, as it can be dry. Try thighs or tenderloins - these are generally more moist.
- Suitable to freeze.
- S* This recipe is suitable on the soft diet if you ensure the vegetables are cooked until tender and can be broken with the side of a fork.

"Very tender, easy to eat."
- Jane, gastric bypass -

"Easy to make, easy to chew and I was satisfied after eating."
- Frances, gastric band -

191

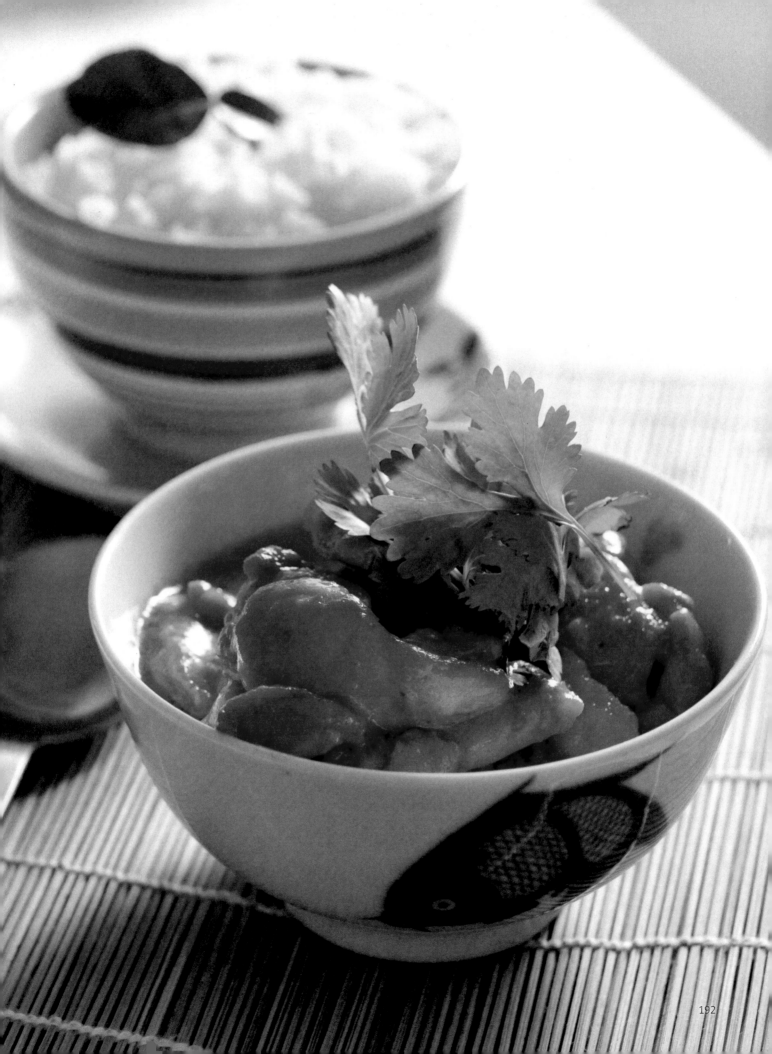

Chicken Schnitzel & Chips

Makes 4 cups

Oil spray

400g chicken tenderloins, trimmed of fat

1 cup buttermilk

Crumb mixture

½ cup breadcrumbs

¼ cup polenta

1 tablespoon parsley, chopped

1 tablespoon Parmesan cheese, finely grated

Chips

2 medium potatoes

1 teaspoon oil

Mixed herbs

If you would enjoy a sauce with your schnitzels, try Yoghurt Dipping Sauce (page 213). For larger appetites (family and friends) consider a vegetable side dish such as Oven Roasted Vegetable Salad (page 36).

Combine ingredients for crumb mixture well. Marinate chicken in buttermilk for about 1 hour. Halve potatoes and cut into thin wedges. Place potatoes, oil and mixed herbs in a plastic bag and mix until potato is well coated. Preheat oven to 200°C. Remove the chicken from the buttermilk and let the excess buttermilk drain from the chicken. Toss in the crumb mixture until well coated. Place chicken and chips on a non-stick baking tray and spray with oil spray. If you don't have a non-stick tray, line a baking tray with baking paper and spray with oil. Bake at 200°C for 15 minutes or until chicken is cooked through.

Nutrition information (per cup): kilojoules 1135, calories 272, protein 23g, fat 12g, saturated fat 3.5g, carbohydrate 17g, fibre 2g.

"Your chicken schnitzels are superb! I've used egg white in recipes like this previously but not buttermilk. It works so well."
- Elaine, gastric band -

"My husband and I really enjoyed this. Very satisfying."
- Terrina, gastric band -

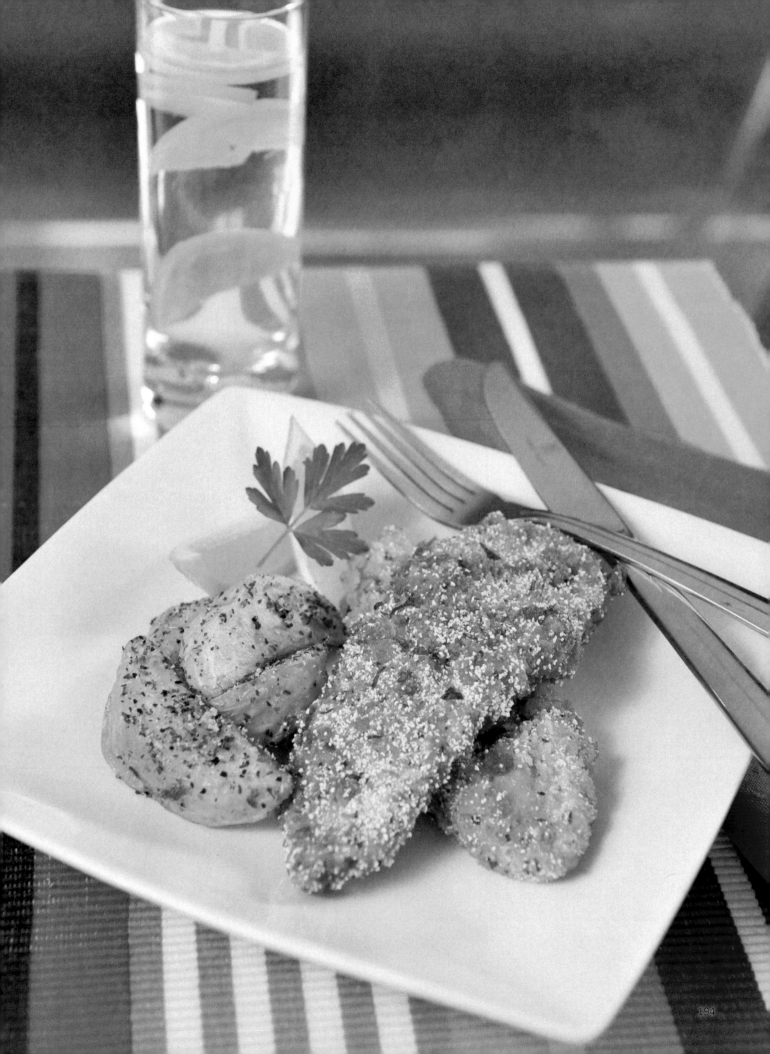

Pumpkin, Spinach & Ricotta Cannelloni (s)

Makes 4 cups

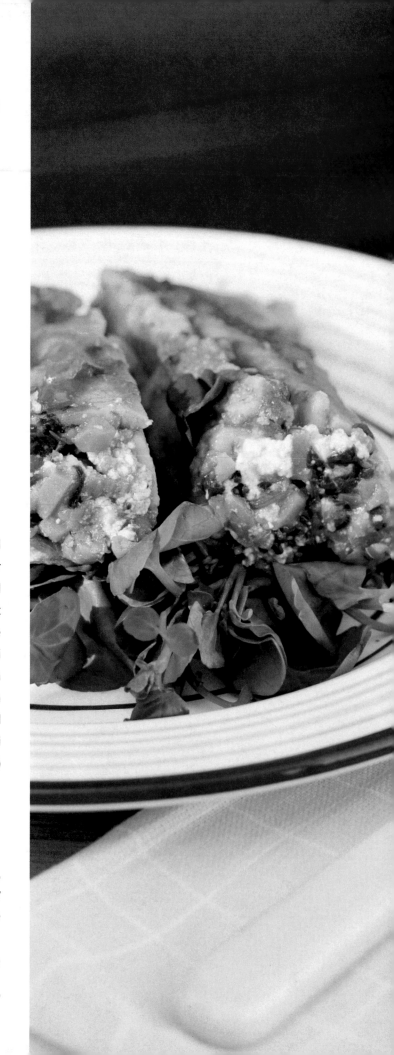

Oil spray

1 cup butternut pumpkin, diced

2 cups chopped spinach or baby spinach

3 garlic cloves

150g low fat ricotta cheese

Handful of basil, finely shredded

1½ cups no added salt tomato pasta sauce

¼ cup dry white wine

2 tablespoons (30g) whey protein isolate powder

1/4 cup water

8 cannelloni tubes

4 tablespoons Parmesan cheese, grated

Preheat oven to 200°C. Spray an oven tray with oil and bake pumpkin and garlic for 10-15 minutes or until tender. Cool slightly then mash the pumpkin and garlic together. Cook spinach in a frying pan until just soft. Mix pumpkin, spinach, ricotta and basil. Fill the cannelloni tubes with the mixture. Place cannelloni in an oven proof dish. Dissolve protein powder in water. Combine dissolved powder, wine and pasta sauce and pour over the cannelloni. Cover and bake approximately 30 minutes, or until cannelloni is cooked. Sprinkle each serve (2 cannelloni tubes) with a tablespoon of grated parmesan.

Nutrition information (per cup): kilojoules 1020, calories 244, protein 18g, fat 7.5g, saturated fat 4g, carbohydrate 23.5g, fibre 2g.

- Larger appetites (family and friends) may enjoy a side salad with this meal, such as a simple green salad.
- Suitable to freeze. Add a little extra pasta sauce if cannelloni becomes dry when reheating.

Mixed Vegetable Pizza

Makes 4 cups

2 small wholemeal pita bread

4 tablespoons no added salt tomato pasta sauce

¼ teaspoon basil

¼ teaspoon oregano

2 mushrooms, sliced

1 tomato, halved and sliced

½ onion, finely sliced

½ capsicum, roasted and diced

½ cup pumpkin, thinly sliced and grilled/roasted

½ cup eggplant, roasted

½ cup zucchini, roasted

1 cup reduced fat mozzarella cheese, grated

1 tablespoon Parmesan cheese, grated

Pre-heat oven to 180°C. Place pita bread on oven trays and spread the pita bread with tomato pasta sauce. Prepare all other toppings, and spread evenly over each pita bread, finishing with the cheese. Bake in the oven for approximately 15 minutes, until the cheese is melted and the bread is crisp.

Nutrition information (per cup or half pizza): kilojoules 930, calories 222, protein 15g, fat 7g, saturated fat 4g, carbohydrate 22g, fibre 4.5g.

Larger appetites (family and friends) would generally need 2 serves (a full pita) and may like their pizza served with a Mushroom Salad (page 44) or simple green salad.

"Love it!"

- Lisa, gastric band -

"The Mixed Vegetable Pizza was very yummy and very filling. You don't feel like you are depriving yourself because it is just like a normal meal."

- Tania, gastric bypass -

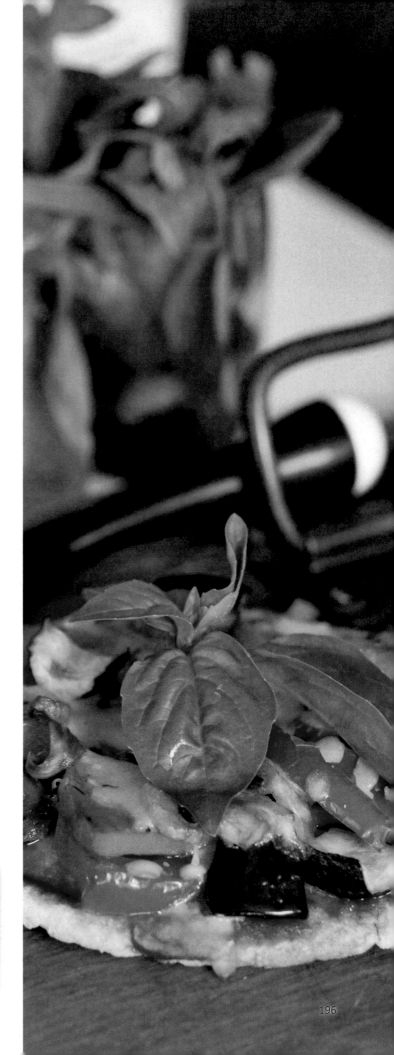

Chicken Curry S*

Makes 4 cups

1 tablespoon canola oil

400g chicken, trimmed of fat, cut into strips
eg. breast, thigh or tenderloin

Juice of 1 lemon

1 onion, thinly sliced

1 clove garlic, crushed

1 cinnamon stick

4 cardamom pods, crushed

4 cloves

½ teaspoon ground cumin

1½ tablespoons ground coriander

½ teaspoon ground ginger

1½ teaspoons turmeric

1 small red chilli, seeded and sliced (or chilli
powder, to taste)

½ cup salt reduced chicken stock

12 dried apricot halves, soaked, drained and cut
into strips or ¼ cup sultanas

1 tablespoon fruit or mango chutney, to serve

½ cup low fat natural yoghurt, to serve

1 cup cauliflower florets, steamed

1 cup broccoli florets, steamed

Sprinkle chicken with lemon juice. Heat oil in a frying pan and stir-fry onions and garlic until onions are soft, but not brown. Add spices and chilli (if desired) and cook, stirring for 4-5 minutes. Add chicken and stir-fry until it is well coated with spices and just white. Add stock and apricots or sultanas and simmer gently for about 10 minutes until chicken is cooked through. Add a squeeze of lemon juice to taste. Remove cinnamon stick and serve topped with yoghurt and a side of steamed cauliflower and broccoli.

Nutrition information (per cup): kilojoules 1120, calories 268, protein 23.5g, fat 13g, saturated fat 3g, carbohydrate 12g, fibre 3g.

- This curry works well with lamb or beef, just simmer a little longer than 10 minutes, until meat is cooked through.
- Suitable to freeze.
- S* This recipe is suitable on the soft diet if you ensure the vegetables are cooked until tender and can be broken with the side of a fork.

"Lovely. Really good flavours. I used thighs, mainly because I tend to tolerate thigh better than breast."
- Sarah, gastric bypass, 2010 -

"Beautiful!"
- Helen, gastric band -

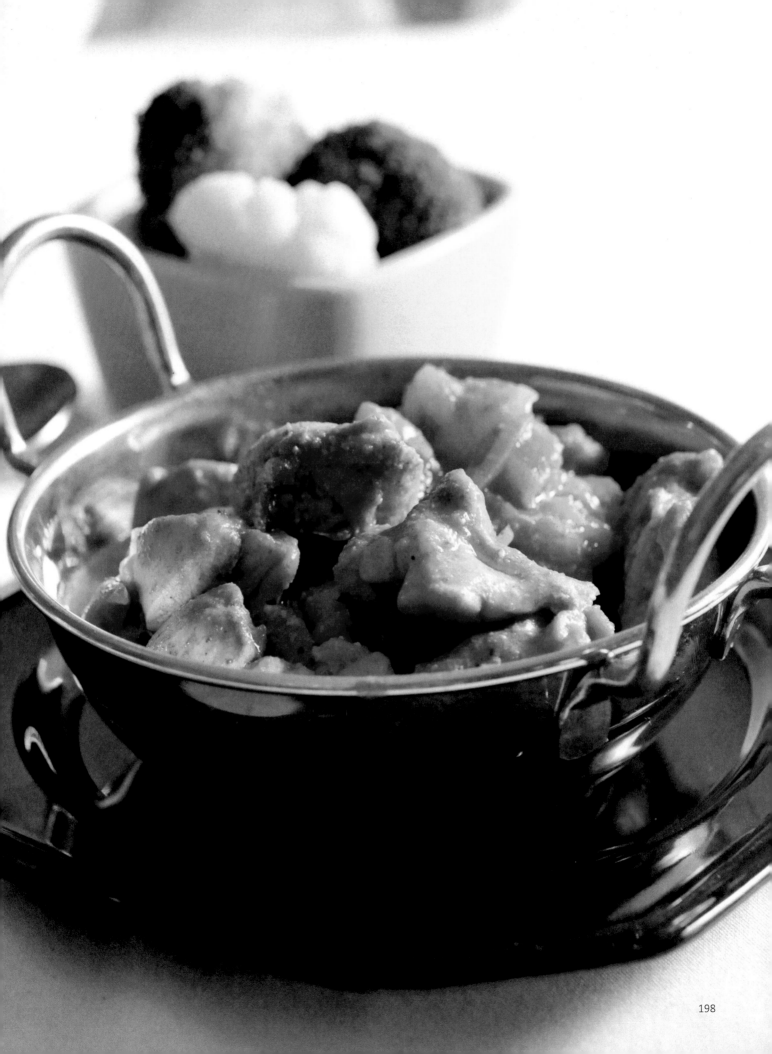

Caesar Salad

Makes 4 cups

2 slices wholegrain/multigrain bread, crust removed

2 teaspoons olive oil

2 cloves garlic, crushed

4 bacon eyes, trimmed of fat, diced

1-2 baby cos lettuces, leaves separated (2 if serving people with larger appetites)

4 eggs

1 tablespoon vinegar

20g Parmesan cheese, shaved

Dressing

2 cloves garlic, crushed

1 tablespoon mustard

1 tablespoon lemon juice

2 anchovies, finely diced

½ cup low fat natural yoghurt

Preheat oven to 180°C. Cut bread into small cubes. Combine oil and garlic in a small bowl. Add bread and toss to coat in oil and garlic. Place bacon and bread in a single layer on oven tray. Toast, uncovered, for approximately 10 minutes. Meanwhile combine ingredients for dressing in screw top jar and shake well. To poach egg, boil 5cm water in a saucepan. Add vinegar. Break eggs into a cup, one at a time, and then gently slide each egg into the saucepan. Allow water to simmer gently for 2-3 minutes until egg white is set. Place lettuce, croutons and bacon in a bowl. Drizzle with dressing and toss gently until well combined. Divide into 4 serves and top each serve with a poached egg. Garnish with Parmesan cheese.

To prevent the egg white spreading in the water whilst poaching, stir the water in the saucepan until it is spinning like a whirlpool, and gently slide an egg into the centre. Eggs will need to be cooked individually using this method.

Nutrition information (per cup): kilojoules 1100, calories 263, protein 21.5g, fat 14g, saturated fat 4.5g, carbohydrate 10.5g, fibre 2g.

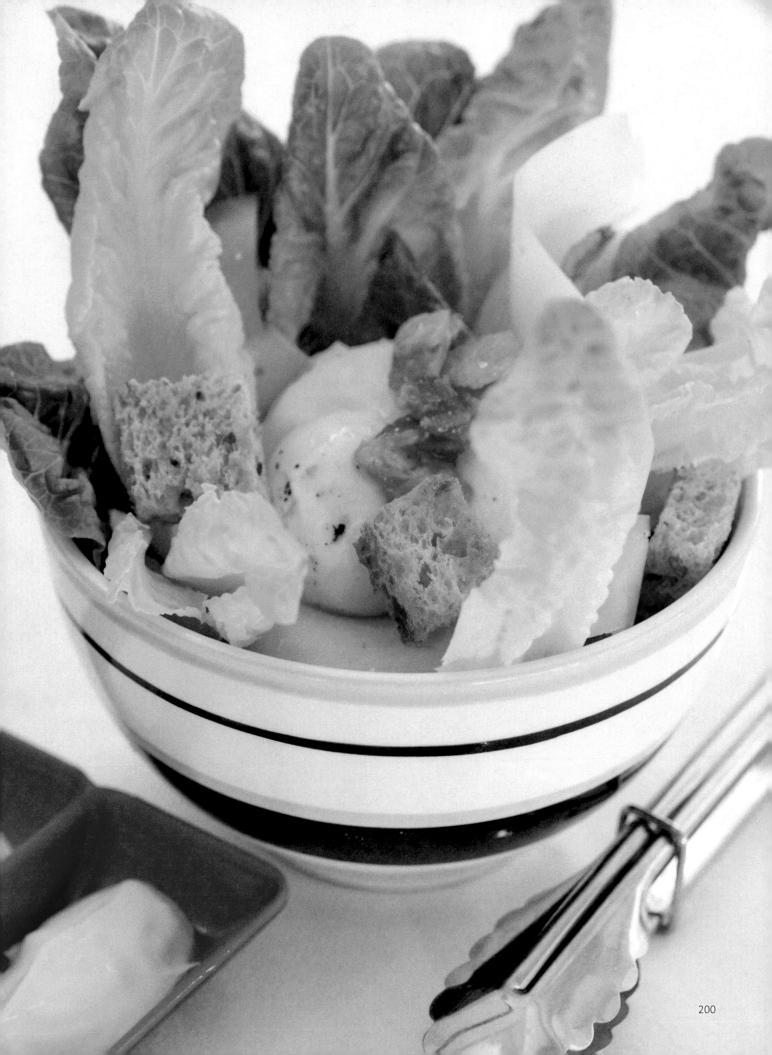

Tofu Stir-fry

Makes 4 cups

1 teaspoon sesame oil

½ onion sliced,

2 cloves garlic, crushed

200g packet Thai flavoured firm tofu

1 small or ½ large red capsicum, sliced

1 bunch bok choy, sliced into strips

½ 230g can bamboo shoots, drained & dried

½ zucchini, halved lengthways and sliced

5 mushrooms, sliced

1 tablespoon oyster sauce

1 teaspoon fish sauce

3 tablespoons tamarind paste

100g udon noodles

Heat oil in a wok over high heat. Add the onion and garlic and stir-fry for 1-2 minutes. Add tofu, capsicum, bok choy, bamboo shoots, zucchini and mushrooms and stir-fry for another 2-3 minutes until bok choy is softening. Add oyster sauce, fish sauce, tamarind paste and noodles. Stir until well combined.

Nutrition information (per cup): kilojoules 685, calories 164, protein 10g, fat 5.5g, saturated fat 1g, carbohydrate 16.5g, fibre 2.5g.

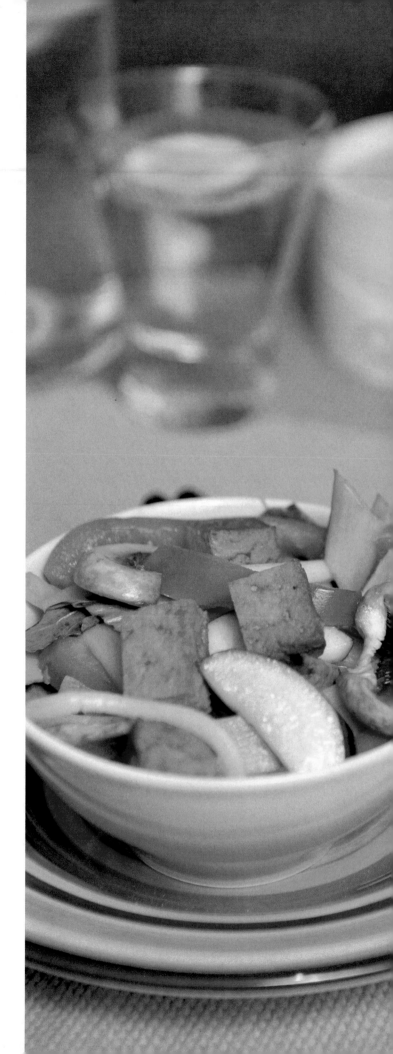

Veal Parmigiana

Makes 4 cups

Oil spray

400g veal leg steaks, trimmed of fat

1 onion, finely diced

2 cloves garlic, crushed

1 cup no added salt, crushed tinned tomatoes

2 tablespoons no added salt tomato paste

2 teapoons balsamic vinegar

1 teaspoon sugar

1 tablespoon fresh basil leaves, shredded

½ large or one small eggplant

¾ cup reduced fat cheese, grated

Heat a frying pan that has been sprayed with oil. Add onion and garlic and cook, stirring until onion is soft. Add tomatoes, tomato paste, vinegar and sugar. Simmer, uncovered, approximately 10 minutes or until sauce thickens, then stir in basil. The sauce can be made a day ahead if desired and refrigerated, covered, overnight. Cut unpeeled eggplant into ½ -1cm slices. Cook in a frying pan or barbeque that has been sprayed with oil until browned both sides. Cook veal one side, turn and top with sauce, eggplant and cheese. Cook until cheese is melted and veal is cooked to the desired tenderness.

Nutrition information (per cup): kilojoules 980, calories 234, protein 29.5g, fat 9g, saturated fat 4g, carbohydrate 6.5g, fibre 2.5g.

- If you have diabetes, serve with a small piece of bread. Larger appetites (family and friends) may also enjoy some bread as a side.
- For home made garlic bread, slice bread, spray with oil, rub with a clove of garlic. Reassemble as a whole, wrap in foil and bake in the oven until warmed through.

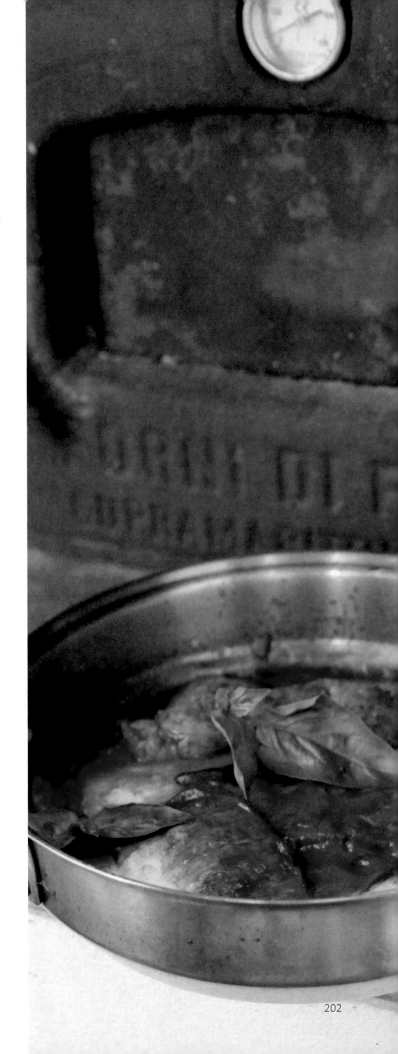

Thai Fish Parcels & Stir-fry Vegetables S*

Makes 4 cups

500g (4 x 125g) fish fillets eg. salmon, barramundi

2 tablespoons sweet chili sauce

2 cloves garlic, minced

3-4 slices lime

Handful fresh coriander

Oil spray

1 carrot, thinly sliced diagonally

1 cup broccoli florets

½ red capsicum, sliced

- If you have diabetes, add a small serve of hokkien or rice noodles to the stir-fry. Larger appetites (family and friends) may also enjoy these as a side dish.
- S* This recipe is suitable on the soft diet if you ensure the vegetables are cooked until tender and can be broken with the side of a fork.

Recipe inspiration courtesy of Sharon, gastric band, 2010.

Preheat oven to 180°C. Place 4 x 30cm squares of baking paper on top of 4 x 30cm squares of foil. Place fish fillets in centre of baking paper. Combine half of the garlic and half of the sweet chili sauce and drizzle over fish. Top with fresh coriander and a slice of lime. Fold into a parcel and bake for about 10-12 minutes then let stand for 5 minutes (fish will continue to cook from residual heat). Meanwhile, heat a frying pan or wok that has been sprayed with oil. Add garlic and cook for about a minute. Add carrot and cook, stirring for 1-2 minutes. Add broccoli and capsicum and cook, stirring for about 5 minutes until veges are cooked but still a little crisp. Drizzle with the remaining sweet chilli sauce and mix well before removing from the pan. Serve fish with stir-fried vegetables.

Nutrition information (per cup): kilojoules 750, calories 179, protein 27g, fat 4g, saturated fat 1g, carbohydrate 7g, fibre 2g.

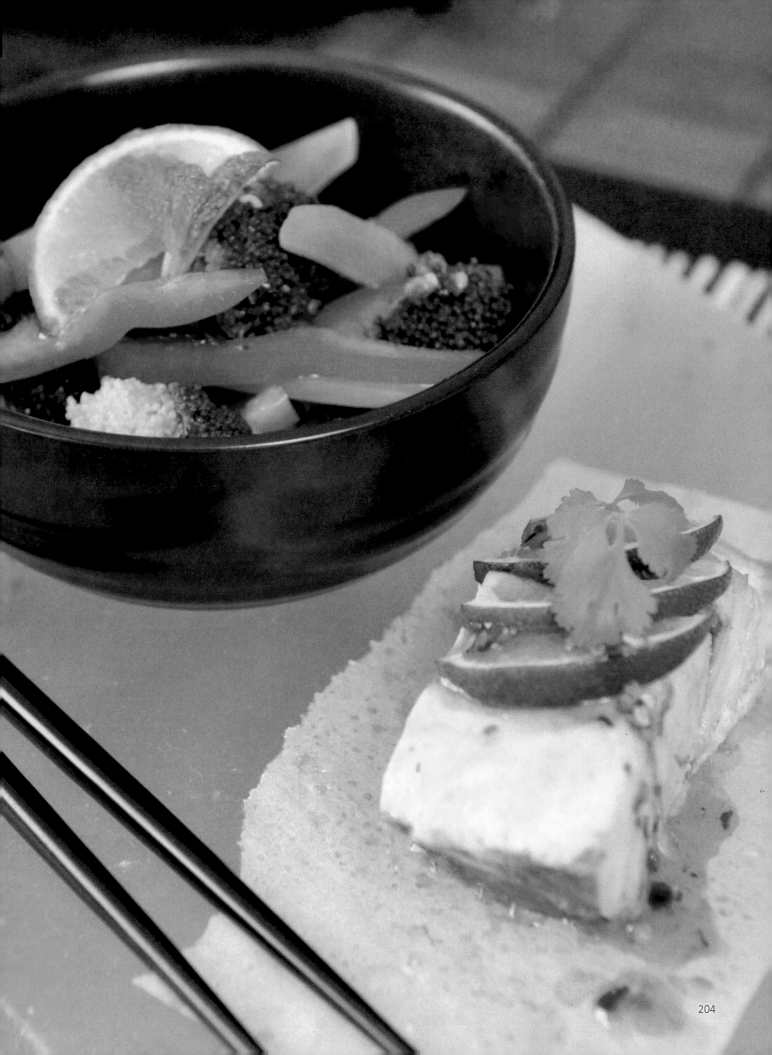

Chicken Satay Cups 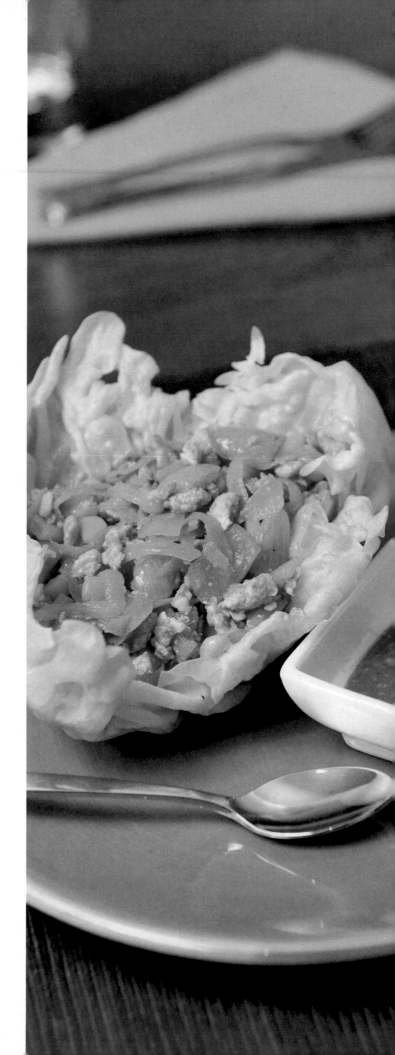 S*

Makes 4 cups

1 teaspoon peanut oil

400g lean chicken mince

⅓ cup mild satay sauce

1 onion, diced

1 carrot, grated

125g can corn kernels, drained

4 iceberg lettuce leaf cups

Heat oil in a wok over medium to high heat. Add onion and mince and stir-fry for about 5 minutes, or until browned, breaking up mince as it cooks. Add satay sauce and stir-fry until well combined. Add carrot and corn and stir-fry for 1 to 2 minutes until carrot is tender. Spoon mixture into lettuce leaf cups to serve.

Nutrition information (per cup): kilojoules 1120, calories 263, protein 21.5g, fat 14.5g, saturated fat 4g, carbohydrate 12g, fibre 2g.

- Prior to cooking, place lettuce leaves in a bowl of iced water for 10 minutes (this makes them crisp). Drain and pat dry.
- The chicken satay filling can be frozen and defrosted to serve in the lettuce cups at a later date.
- S* This recipe is suitable on the soft diet if you serve without the lettuce.

Recipe suggestion courtesy of Mercy Bariatrics.

Italian Chicken Pasta

Makes 4 cups

Oil Spray

300g skinless chicken, trimmed of fat and diced eg. breast, tenderloin, thigh

½ onion, diced

2 cloves garlic, minced

1 cup no added salt, chopped tinned tomatoes

1 cup mushrooms, sliced

2 tablespoons balsamic vinegar

1 teaspoon basil

1 teaspoon oregano

½ teaspoon rosemary

2 tablespoons no added salt tomato paste

1 cup dry pasta eg. small spirals or shells

4 tablespoons Parmesan cheese

Heat a frying pan that has been sprayed with oil. Add onion, garlic and mushrooms and cook for approximately 5 minutes over low heat. Add chicken and cook over medium to high heat until no longer pink. Add tomatoes, paste, vinegar and herbs to the mixture. Mix well, cover and simmer over medium-low heat for 20 minutes. As sauce is simmering, cook pasta according to directions on packet. Combine with sauce and sprinkle with Parmesan to serve.

Nutrition information (per cup): kilojoules 1010, calories 242, protein 20.5g, fat 10g, saturated fat 3.5g, carbohydrate 15.5g, fibre 3g.

Larger appetites (family and friends) may enjoy a side salad with this meal, such as a simple green salad.

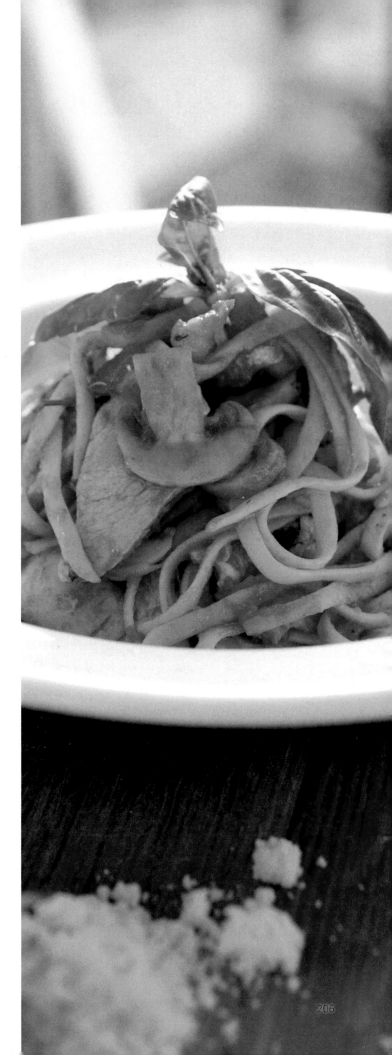

Slow Cooked Lamb Curry S*

Makes 4 cups

Oil spray

450g lamb, trimmed of fat, diced into cubes

1 onion, sliced

1 tablespoon flour

2 cloves garlic, crushed

¼ teaspoon cumin seeds

1 cup salt reduced chicken stock

1 tablespoon sweet chutney

1 tablespoon curry powder (or to taste)

1 tablespoon sultanas

1 teaspoon lemon zest

½ cup sweet potato, diced

1 cup cauliflower, chopped

¼ cup frozen peas

¼ cup low fat natural yogurt

8 mini Pappadums

Pre-heat oven to 150°C. Spray a casserole dish with oil spray. Heat a large saucepan that has been sprayed with oil. Sauté the onion and garlic until softened. Stir in the curry powder and cumin seeds and cook, stirring, until the spices become fragrant. Toss the lamb in the flour, add lamb to the saucepan and brown a little. Pour in the chicken stock. Add the chutney, sultanas and lemon zest. Bring to the boil then add the sweet potato and cauliflower. Stir to combine then remove from the heat. Pour into the casserole dish, cover and place in oven and cook for 1½ hours, gently stirring a couple of times during cooking. After 1½ hours stir through the frozen peas and continue to cook for another 30 minutes, uncovered. At this stage some of the meat and veggies may seem dry, but this is only on the surface. Remove from the oven and stir through the yoghurt.

Place the pappadums in a circle in the microwave and cook on high for 40-60 seconds until they are crisp. Serve the curry with 2 mini pappadums per person and garnish with a teaspoon of yogurt.

Nutrition information (per cup): kilojoules 1245, calories 298, protein 28g, fat 9g, saturated fat 3.5g, carbohydrate 23g, fibre 5g.

- Suitable to freeze.
- S* This recipe is suitable on the soft diet if you ensure the vegetables are cooked until tender and can be broken with the side of a fork.
- Alternatively, you can omit the oil spray and combine the next 10 ingredients in a slow cooker and cook for approximately 8 hours. It is best to add the vegetables for the last 1-2 hours, so they don't become too soft. If using this method, you will only need 1/2 cup of stock, not the full cup.

> "I love it! It was filling and the pappadums added a nice crunchy texture."
>
> - Sharon, gastric band -

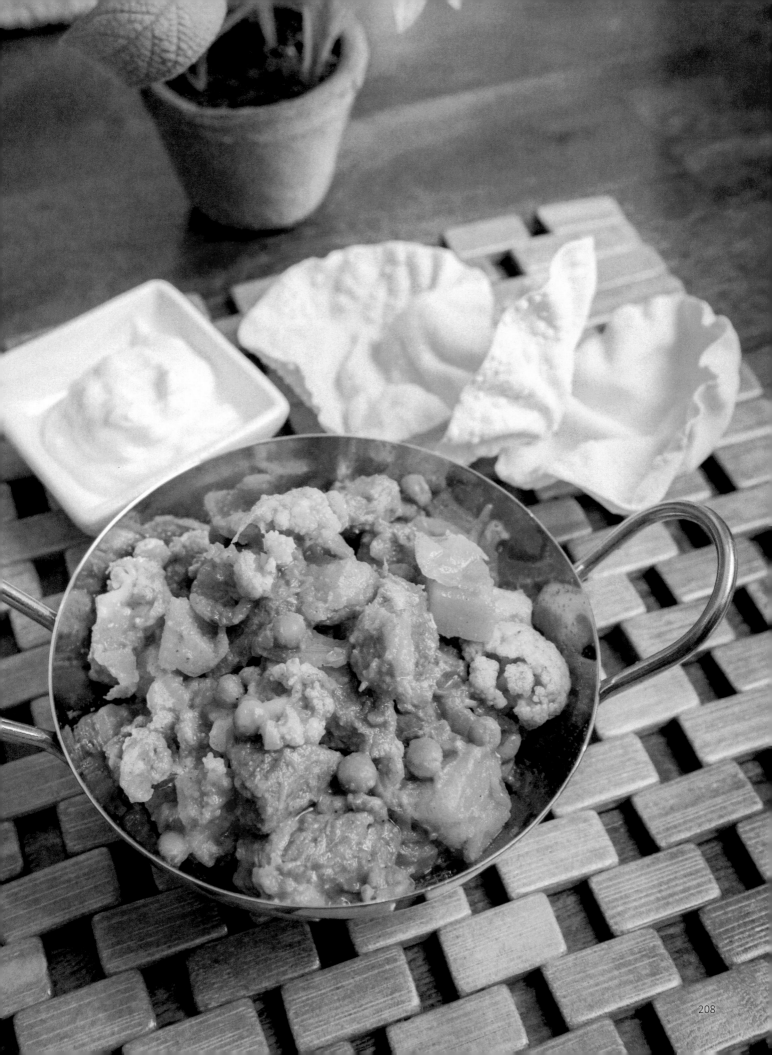

Creamy Chicken & Sweet Potato Casserole s*

Makes 4 cups

2 teaspoons olive oil

400g skinless chicken, trimmed of fat, diced eg. breast, thigh or tenderloin

1 small fennel bulb, trimmed, thinly sliced

Sprinkle of dried thyme

2 cloves garlic, crushed

¼ cup dry white wine

1 tablespoon wholegrain mustard

1½ cups sweet potato, peeled and chopped

½ cup salt reduced chicken stock

¼ cup Philadephia® Cream for Cooking Extra Light

Cornflour, as required

s* This recipe is suitable on the soft diet if you ensure the vegetables are cooked until tender and can be broken with the side of a fork.

Heat oil in a frying pan over medium-high heat. Add chicken in batches and cook, stirring for a few minutes until slightly golden. Remove chicken from frying pan and set aside. Add fennel, thyme and garlic to pan. Cook, stirring, for 5 minutes or until soft. Add wine and mustard and cook for 3 minutes. Add sweet potato and stock and bring to the boil. Return chicken to the pan. Cover and reduce heat to low. Simmer for 30 minutes. Add Philadephia® cream and cook, stirring, for a further 5 minutes but do not boil. If sauce is thin and runny when ready to serve, dissolve 1 teaspoon of cornflour in 1-2 teaspoons of water and stir well to make a paste. Add paste to pan and combine well. If mixture remains runny, repeat with another 1-2 teaspoons of cornflour until sauce is a creamier texture. Season with pepper to serve.

Nutrition information (per cup): kilojoules 1060, calories 254, protein 21.5g, fat 11.5g, saturated fat 3.5g, carbohydrate 13.5g, fibre 3g.

Recipe suggestion courtesy of Mercy Bariatrics.

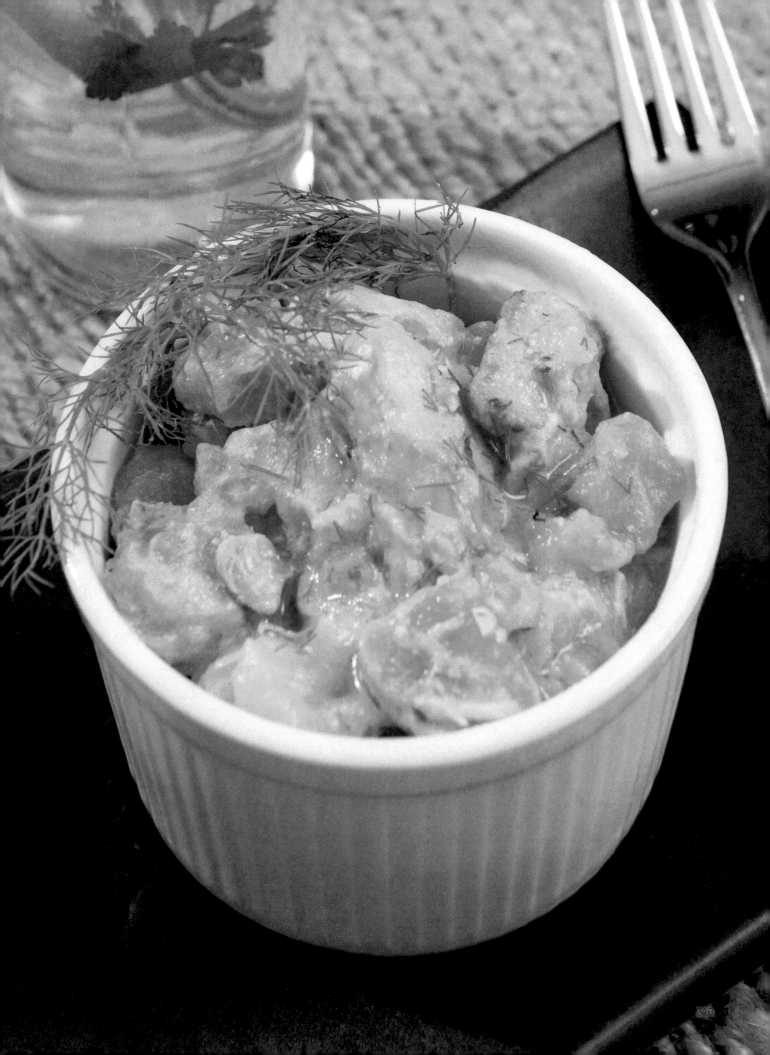

Veal Saltimbocca

Makes 4 cups

Oil spray

400g thin veal steaks, halved

8 sage leaves or 1-2 teaspoons dried sage

8 slices lean shaved ham

⅓ cup white wine

½ cup Philadephia® Cream for Cooking Extra Light

2 teaspoons mustard

1 small head broccoli, steamed

Heat a frying pan that has been sprayed with oil. Top each piece of veal with 1 sage leaf (or a sprinkle of sage) and 1 slice of ham. Ensure the pan is hot before adding veal, and don't overcrowd the pan or the veal will stew. Add the veal, ham side down, and cook for 1½ minutes. Turn and cook for 1 minute. Transfer to a plate and cover with foil to keep warm. Add the wine to the pan and cook for 30 seconds. Add the cooking cream and mustard. Cook, stirring, for 2 minutes or until the sauce thickens. Pour sauce over veal steaks and serve with steamed broccoli.

Nutrition information (per cup): kilojoules 965, calories 231, protein 31g, fat 6.5g, saturated fat 2g, carbohydrate 6g, fibre 5g.

- If you have diabetes, serve with some steamed or oven baked sweet potato.
- If thin veal steaks are not available, beat them with a meat mallet to make them thinner.

> "This is a really good meal when you want something fast. I find fresh sage leaves to be much better than dried if you can get them. The sauce is a great accompaniment. I threw some finely chopped parsley into the sauce just before serving for colour and flavour."
>
> - Robyn, gastric bypass -

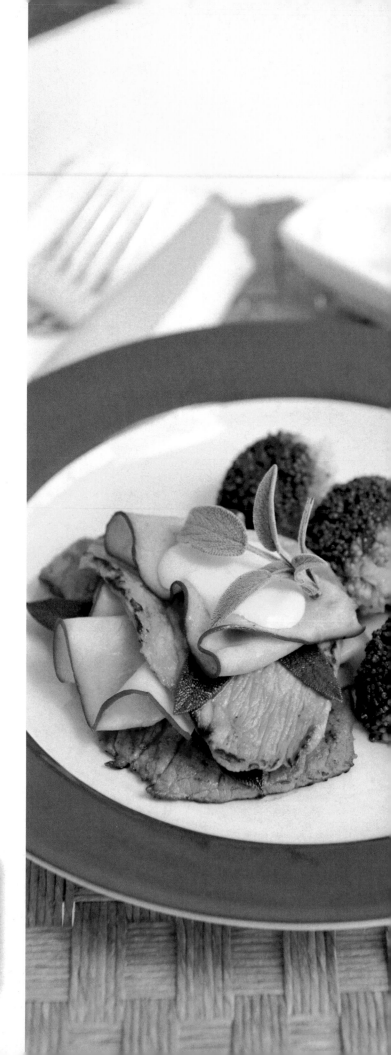

Ingredients: Legumes

Chickpeas

Makes approximately 4 cups

1½ cups chickpeas, soaked* and drained

4 cups water

Place the chickpeas in a saucepan and add the water. Bring mixture to the boil, then boil steadily, uncovered, for 10 minutes. Reduce the heat and simmer the beans for 55-60 minutes or until tender. Drain the excess liquid.

Kidney beans

Makes approximately 4 cups

2 cups red kidney beans, soaked* and drained

4 cups water

Place the red kidney beans in a saucepan and add the water. Bring mixture to the boil, then boil steadily, uncovered, for 10 minutes. Reduce the heat and simmer the beans for 45-60 minutes or until tender. Drain the excess liquid.

Red lentils

Makes approximately 4 cups

2 cups red split lentils

2 cups water

Place the lentils in a container and rinse twice with plenty of cold water to remove dust and grit. Cover with water and stand for 1 hour. Drain the lentils and place in a saucepan and just cover with cold water. Bring the water to the boil and boil for 5 minutes, removing any scum that rises to the top of the water. Reduce the heat and simmer the lentils until they are tender, about 10-15 minutes.

*Dried beans and chickpeas must be soaked prior to cooking. Soak overnight in a large bowl covered with water. If a quick method is preferred, place in a large saucepan and add cold water to cover. Bring to the boil, cover the saucepan and cook for 2 minutes. Remove from heat and let stand for 1 hour.

If you choose to use canned varieties of beans, chickpeas or lentils, drain all fluid and rinse well prior to use.

Ingredients: Dips, Spreads & Sauces

Hummus

2½ cups chickpeas

½ cup tahini

½ cup lemon juice to taste

½ cup water

1 clove garlic

Soak dried chickpeas for 48 hours, then boil for about 4 hours or until very mushy. Strain and place in food processor. Add tahini, garlic (crushed), water and lemon. Puree until smooth.

Serve sprinkled with paprika.

Tzatziki

1kg low fat natural yoghurt

2 Lebanese cucumbers, grated

1-2 cloves garlic, crushed

Squeeze of lemon juice, to taste

Line a sieve with a clean Chux® or muslin cloth and strain the yoghurt overnight. Do the same for the cucumber. Combine strained yoghurt, cucumber, lemon juice and garlic and mix well.

Yoghurt dipping sauce

Makes enough for 4 to use as a sauce

½ cup low fat natural yoghurt

2 tablespoons sweet chilli sauce

1 clove garlic, crushed

½ tablespoon fresh parsley, chopped

Combine ingredients well.

Spiced yoghurt

½ cup low fat natural yoghurt

2 teaspoons lemon juice

1 teaspoon ground cumin

To make yoghurt, combine all ingredients in small bowl. This is best made ahead. Cover and refrigerate 1 hour or overnight.

Ingredients: Stocks

Beef stock

1½kg beef bones, rinsed and fat removed

2½L water (or enough to cover bones)

1 carrot, chopped

1 onion, chopped

2 stalks celery, chopped

1 teaspoon black peppercorns

3 sprigs parsley

1 sprig fresh thyme

1 bay leaf

Place bones and water into saucepan. Bring slowly to the boil. Add vegetables and herbs and simmer for 2 hours. Strain through a sieve and chill. Skim fat from the surface before using. Keep in refrigerator. May be frozen.

Fish stock

250g fish bones and head

3 cups cold water

1 onion, chopped

1 stalk celery, chopped

1 slice lemon

3 parsley sprigs

2 peppercorns

Wash bones and place in saucepan with water. Bring slowly to the boil. Add vegetables and flavourings, simmer* for 30 minutes. Strain through a fine sieve or cheesecloth.

*For the best flavour, fish stock must be simmered, never boiled.

Vegetable stock

Follow recipe for Beef Stock, omitting the beef bones. Use a variety of vegetables. Trimmings such as celery tops, Brussels sprout leaves, mushroom peelings, tomato and onion skins can be used. Simmer for 1 hour.

Chicken stock

Follow recipe for Beef Stock (above). Use chicken bones and giblets instead of beef. Cook for 1 hour.

Troubleshooting and Common Complaints

Troubleshooting and Common Complaints

For those considering weight loss surgery, this chapter may seem a little confronting. That is not the intent. It is important to remember that everyone has a different experience following surgery. Most people will be unlikely to experience the potential problems discussed in this chapter, but for those who do, this section may be useful. Skim over the headings in this section, then come back and read more if you encounter any of the problems listed during your journey.

Regurgitation

Regurgitation can occur after any form of weight loss surgery. It is thought to be most common in the early stages following surgery as you are adapting to the correct eating technique. Your surgical team may use the words interchangeably, but regurgitation is different from vomiting. Vomiting is when food has reached the stomach and is rejected. Regurgitation is when food is rejected before entering the stomach.

If you have trouble tolerating particular foods in the early stages following surgery, don't give up trying them. Food aversions and poor tolerance are more common in the early stages until the correct way of eating becomes a habit. Stringy, tough or doughy foods may be hard to tolerate long term, so if they continue to be a problem, avoid them.

Long term issues with regurgitation are often due to:

- eating too quickly
- not chewing food well enough
- eating food that is difficult to chew to a smooth texture – tough, stringy or doughy foods
- taking bites of food that are too big
- eating too much at one time
- for those with a gastric band, being in the red zone.

If you regularly regurgitate food you first need to pay attention to your eating technique. Read more on the correct eating technique in the *Food Fundamentals Following Weight Loss Surgery* chapter (page 98). If there is no change, contact your support team to discuss what is happening.

Regurgitation and over inflated gastric bands

There is a mistaken perception among those with a gastric band that regurgitation is normal. Regular regurgitation is not normal. It is a sign of one or more of the problems previously listed, or an over inflated, or tight gastric band.

Unfortunately, along with the belief that regurgitation is normal, is the belief that a tighter band will result in faster and greater weight loss. This is also incorrect. A band that is too tight leads to poor eating behaviour and unpleasant side effects. When the band is too tight many people find it difficult to lose weight. One reason for this is that the food that is easy to eat is not healthy food. The soft, slippery, easy to chew or liquid foods are often high in fat and/or sugar and therefore high in energy (calories or kilojoules). Eating high-energy foods and fluids will ultimately result in weight regain.

If a gastric band is tight for an extended time it can lead to medical complications. As well as more regular regurgitation, a tight band can put too much pressure on the oesophagus and the stomach, therefore affecting their normal function. Some of the side effects can be quite serious and not reversible. These will generally need to be treated with further surgery.

No matter what you may have heard, a tighter band is not a way to fast track healthy weight loss.

Refer to the zone chart for more information (page 12).

A gastric band is a tool in your weight loss journey to help you feel satisfied on less food, not to stop you eating or make eating difficult or uncomfortable.

Frothy regurgitation

Some people with a gastric band will find the first bite or two of food feels as if it sticks causing regurgitation of a frothy, mucous like substance. Generally, once this mucous is cleared (by regurgitation) you can eat normally.

Whilst there are no scientific studies to explain this, it is thought that fibres left from the previous meal may gather across the opening of the band (similar to the fibres that remain across the drain of the sink after you wash the dishes). As we swallow saliva, some will drain through and some will catch on the fibres. This forms a 'plug' that then catches the first bite or two of food at the next meal.

This can be managed by having a drink before starting the meal to help clear any mucous and lubricate the oesophagus and stomach ready for food. Warm fluid may be most effective, or sipping some fluid slowly to soften the mucous, then some fluid quickly to flush the mucous past the band. Be aware that these techniques may help to flush mucous past the band, or they may cause it to be regurgitated. Experiment with these strategies to see what suits you best. Also refer to the zone chart (page 12) to check you have not slipped into the red zone.

Whilst there are no studies to explain it, some people with a sleeve gastrectomy will experience frothy regurgitation. It may be more common in those with reflux, or after overeating. This should be discussed with your team. Some people also experience regurgitation of excess saliva after gastric bypass surgery. This mostly occurs in the mornings in the first few months following surgery. Drinking fluids, particularly warm fluids, helps thin the saliva and alleviates the symptoms.

Shoulder tip pain

Shoulder tip pain is a common complaint after laparoscopic (keyhole) surgery. It may last anywhere from two to three days after surgery, up to five weeks or more. Several factors have been thought to contribute to shoulder tip pain including the effect of gas used to create space in the stomach cavity during surgery, irritation or damage to the diaphragm or even movement of the shoulder during surgery.

Some people find simple pain relief such as paracetamol or codeine will relieve the pain a little. Some find applying heat to the area makes them more comfortable. Others will feel better getting out of bed and walking around to get rid of the trapped gas rather than lying down.

If you are troubled by ongoing shoulder tip pain, discuss with your surgical team.

Reflux/indigestion

Reflux or indigestion can occur after all forms of weight loss surgery, however it is likely to have a different cause with each surgery. If you experience these symptoms you should always discuss it with your surgical team.

If suffering from reflux or indigestion, check the following:

- Are you eating and drinking slowly? Try slowing down a little more and see if that helps.
- Are you eating too much?
- Are you eating and drinking at the same time, overfilling a sleeve or a small pouch after bypass?
- Are you sitting upright when eating? Slouching or reclining may worsen the problem.
- Are you eating too close to going to bed? Try to remain upright longer after eating.

Some people will be discharged from hospital with anti-reflux medication. If this occurs you should continue to take the medication for the time period your surgical team recommends.

Poor food tolerance

An Australian study from The St George Upper GI Clinic found that food tolerance and satisfaction with eating is lower for those with a gastric band compared with gastric bypass or sleeve gastrectomy. The study found common problem foods for those with a gastric band include red or white meat, bread, salad vegetables, rice and pasta. Some people who have had sleeve gastrectomy or gastric bypass also reported difficulty eating these foods, but it was far less common than among those with a gastric band.

In her book, *Portion Perfection for Bands and Sleeves,* Amanda Clark, Advanced Accredited Practising Dietitian reports that her own research has found approximately 60% of people with a gastric band find white bread and meat difficult to tolerate. However, this means that about one in three people with a band have no problems tolerating these foods.

Some people will undergo different surgeries in the course of their weight loss journey. It is important to be aware that having difficulty tolerating particular foods with one surgery may not mean it will occur with subsequent surgeries.

In summary, tolerance of foods after each surgery type is very individual and can only be found through trial and error.

Tolerance of all foods can be improved by following the correct eating technique as discussed in the *Food Fundamentals Following Weight Loss Surgery* chapter (page 98). However, there are lots of hints and tips on the following page that can help if you experience problems with any particular foods.

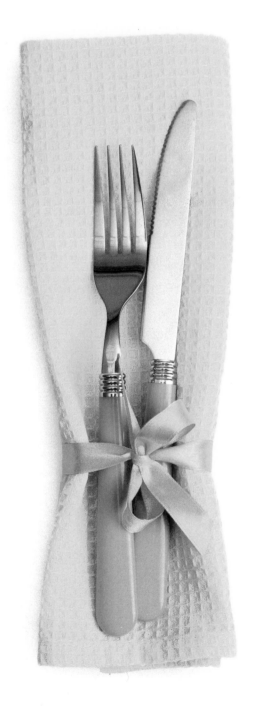

IMPROVING FOOD TOLERANCE

Bread, Cereals, Rice, Pasta and Noodles*

- Don't avoid bread just because someone else who has had surgery told you they can't eat it. Everyone has a different experience so don't be afraid to try.
- Wholegrain/multigrain breads are often easier to tolerate than white or wholemeal.
- Try toasted bread rather than fresh. Remove crusts and see if that helps. Allow the toast to go cold and see if that makes it easier to chew well.
- Cut bread or sandwiches into nine pieces rather than two or four – smaller pieces will help you nibble and take smaller bites.
- Some find wraps more comfortable than sandwich bread – try mountain bread, wraps, tortilla wraps or thin pita breads.
- If bread remains uncomfortable to eat even when taking care with your eating technique, try wholegrain/multigrain crackers. Choose the grainy, denser options such as Vita-weat® or Ryvita®. Limit Cruskits®, rice crackers, rice cakes or Corn Thins® as these will chew up easily, making them easy to overeat. They are also less likely to keep you feeling satisfied.
- Smaller pasta shapes may be easier to eat. It is hard to control the bite size of pasta like fettuccini and spaghetti when it is wound around your fork. Cut these into smaller pieces or try smaller shapes such as penne or spirali that cut into small pieces more easily.
- Experiment with cooking pasta for different lengths of time. Some may find it is easier to eat if overcooked.
- Experiment with different varieties of rice. Some tend to go gluggy or sticky when cooked, whereas others stay separate.
- Serve pasta and rice differently. Avoid serving these as the main component of the meal. Rather than a bed of rice or pasta covering the plate or bottom of the bowl, make these no more than one quarter of the meal. Alternatively, just mix a small amount of rice or pasta through your dish.

In the early stages following sleeve gastrectomy and gastric bypass, bread, pasta and rice can swell in the new, smaller stomach and cause pain and discomfort. These foods can interfere with the intake of protein-containing foods, which are important to help your recovery. If you have diabetes, it is important to include some carbohydrate-containing foods. However, legumes, milk and milk products may be more comfortable to eat and will also provide you with protein. If you are unsure about your intake of these foods or your individual carbohydrate needs, speak with your dietitian.

Fruit

- If you tend to take large bites from pieces of fruit, slice or dice into smaller pieces.
- Slice harder fruits like apples into thin pieces to ensure the skin is broken up. Nibble the thin slices rather than taking big bites. If they still cause problems, grate them.
- Thoroughly remove pith from oranges and mandarins.
- Depending on the variety or ripeness of fruit, skins may vary in toughness. Experiment with different varieties at different times of the season.

IMPROVING FOOD TOLERANCE

Vegetables*

- Always shred lettuce on your plate, like it is shredded at sandwich bars.
- Avoiding folding lettuce leaves into a 'parcel' to get it on your fork – this 'parcel' can open out again once swallowed.
- Try different varieties of lettuce. Whilst iceberg may be easier for some, gourmet lettuce varieties may suit others.
- Try baby spinach or rocket as an alternative to lettuce. You can also remove the stems on these if you find them uncomfortable.
- If lettuce is not comfortable to eat, try other salad vegetables to add a fresh texture – mung bean sprouts, alfalfa, bean shoots or snow pea sprouts.
- Slice tomatoes, cucumber and capsicums thinly to break the skins into smaller pieces.
- Remove strings from snow peas and celery.
- If you find salad vegetables such as raw carrot or cucumber tricky to eat, try grating them.

*In the early stages following sleeve gastrectomy or gastric bypass, be careful not to fill up on these foods. Always eat protein-containing foods first.

Meat and Meat Alternatives

- Cut all meat into five-cent piece size bites.
- Cut meat across the grain to break the meat fibres.
- To slice meat thinly for stir-fries, slice whilst still partly frozen.
- Marinades help tenderise meat, particularly those with an acidic ingredient eg. vinegar, wine, lemon or lime juice.
- Choose better cuts of red meat that are more likely to be tender. You will be eating less, so the expense will even out.
- Choose more moist cuts of chicken. Thighs and tenderloins tend to be more moist and tender when cooked than chicken breast.
- Avoid overcooking meat. Tough, stringy or dry meat is very difficult to tolerate. Rare meat is often easiest to eat.
- Try slow cooking meats. Slow cookers work well, however, you can achieve similar results by cooking casseroles on the stove or in the oven on low heat for several hours.
- Slice meat across the grain into thin stir-fry strips. Dissolve one quarter of a teaspoon of bicarb soda in three tablespoons of water (for 500g meat – adjust if using less). Massage into the meat and marinate for a minimum of three to four hours before stir-frying. This will help tenderise meat.
- Avoid reheating leftover meats unless they are in a sauce/gravy. Slow cooked casseroles and stews are fine to reheat.
- Overcooked seafood can be rubbery. Take care with squid and octopus. If you find these difficult to cook just right, opt for prawns or scallops.

Breakfast

Whilst eating breakfast has not specifically been studied after weight loss surgery, wider research has found breakfast can improve mental performance, reduce fatigue and improve eating habits by reducing snacking during the day. Reflect on your habits. If you skip breakfast do you get hungry mid morning? Are you prepared with a healthy snack or do you grab whatever is available in the lunch room, vending machine or service station? This is a common pitfall of breakfast skippers.

Unfortunately some people with a gastric band report that breakfast is difficult to eat. There are no scientific studies to indicate why this is so, however it is a common phenomenon. One theory is that when we are laying down overnight, body fluids accumulate in the upper part of the abdomen, which may cause a sensation that the band is tighter. Following are a range of potential reasons why breakfast may be harder to eat, each with a suggested solution:

- Are you experiencing frothy regurgitation as described earlier in this chapter? Try the suggested drinking techniques to loosen the mucous.
- Are you eating late at night? Are you eating larger serves at night? Check that your meal sizes are similar and food is spread fairly evenly across the day.
- Did you have food stick and/or regurgitate food the night before? This can cause some swelling of the stomach near the band, making it harder to tolerate food the next time you try to eat.
- Have you always skipped breakfast and just find it hard to change your habits?
- Is your band too tight? Refer to the zone chart.

If none of the above is relevant to you, you may just need to have breakfast a little later when you feel ready. Or you may find a softer or smaller breakfast is enough. A piece of fruit or tub of low fat yoghurt may be all you need. Whilst it is important to focus on solid food as often as possible to get the maximum satisfaction from your food, you may find liquid is all you can manage. The *Smoothies & Soups* (from page 58) has some great tasting, nutritious smoothies you could try for breakfast if fluid is all you tolerate.

Meals should not be skipped totally, as it is then difficult to obtain adequate nutrition during the rest of the day. This is particularly so for those who have had sleeve gastrectomy and gastric bypass surgery.

Dumping syndrome

Dumping syndrome is a common side effect following gastric bypass surgery. One report states that 50-70% of patients will experience dumping syndrome in the early stages after surgery, however, these symptoms will often subside after 15-18 months. Dumping syndrome has also been reported after sleeve gastrectomy. Dumping syndrome usually occurs after making poor food choices, particularly those high in sugar. This can include foods high in natural sugar such as fruit juice.

Dumping syndrome can occur at different times after eating. Early dumping occurs within 10-30 minutes of eating. As food spends less time in the upper part of the digestive system, undigested food parts pass quickly into the lower bowel, causing an influx of fluid into the bowel to try and dilute the food, stretching the bowel and making it contract. This can cause symptoms such as nausea, bloating, abdominal cramps and diarrhoea. Late dumping occurs one to three hours after eating due to low blood glucose (sugar) levels caused by an oversupply of insulin. People experience a drop in blood pressure and increased heart rate, which causes flushing, dizziness, palpitations and an intense feeling of wanting to lie down.

Dumping syndrome is not life threatening. It can be managed by making good food choices and avoiding problem foods, particularly foods and drinks high in sugar such as soft drink, cordial, lollies or sugary desserts like pavlova. If you have ongoing problems with dumping syndrome, discuss this with your dietitian. You may need help reading food labels to learn to identify problem foods. Separating food and fluid, spreading your food intake evenly over the day and choosing low GI foods can also assist.

Reactive Hypoglycemia

Whilst dumping syndrome has long been a recognised complication of weight loss surgery, particularly gastric bypass surgery, in recent years a more severe form of hypoglycemia, reactive hypoglycemia, has become apparent. Where dumping syndrome occurs in the period soon after surgery and improves with time, reactive hypoglycemia can arise later, usually more than one year after surgery.

The key difference between dumping syndrome (which does involve a form of hypoglycemia) and reactive hypoglycaemia is that there is a shortage of glucose to the brain, which can affect the function of neurons and alter brain function. This does not occur in dumping syndrome. Common symptoms of hypoglycemia (in both dumping syndrome and reactive hypoglycaemia) include sweating, shakiness, increased heart rate, anxiety and a feeling of hunger. However, the additional symptoms of reactive hypoglycaemia that are related to brain function include weakness, tiredness, or dizziness, inappropriate behavior which is sometimes mistaken for being under the influence of alcohol, difficulty with concentration, confusion and blurred vision.

Knowing the difference between dumping syndrome and reactive hypoglycaemia can be tricky, however if you have concerns you should discuss them with your team.

Most people with dumping syndrome will find symptoms improve with dietary modification to include small, frequent meals and reducing their carbohydrate intake, particularly sugar. Reactive hypoglycaemia may also be improved with smaller, more frequent meals and an emphasis on low glycemic index foods. However, reactive hypoglycemia does not always respond as well to dietary modification. In both cases medication may be needed hence it is essential to discuss with your team.

Dehydration

Following sleeve gastrectomy and gastric bypass surgeries, the new, smaller stomach simply does not allow you to fit the amount of food or fluid you did prior to surgery, making it harder to drink enough fluid. It is also recommended not to eat and drink at the same time after these surgeries, which reduces the time available for drinking.

After all forms of weight loss surgery, make it a habit to sip fluids throughout the day. Remind yourself to drink often; carry a water bottle with you, keep a jug of water on your desk at work or in a place where you walk past it often at home. If you struggle to drink enough fluid in winter, try warm water with a slice of lemon or herbal teas to warm you up. Set a target to drink at least 1500mL (1½L) of fluid daily.

Dehydration can also occur due to regurgitation or vomiting, hence must be avoided where possible. If this is occurring, speak to your support team.

Constipation or diarrhoea

After weight loss surgery, many people will develop a new bowel habit. For some they will need to use their bowels more often and for some they will need to use them less often. In the early post surgery stages when your diet is mainly fluid or pureed food, you may find your bowels to behave differently, often to one extreme or the other. Over time, this generally does settle, however it may be some weeks after you are back eating 'normal' food.

Diarrhoea is not an expected symptom of gastric band, gastric bypass or sleeve gastrectomy surgeries. Some people will have diarrhoea after gastric bypass or sleeve gastrectomy as a result of dumping syndrome. Taking control of dumping syndrome can help to prevent diarrhoea.

Constipation can occur after all forms of weight loss surgery due to a reduced intake of both fibre and/or fluid. It is particularly common in people who limit or avoid high fibre foods such as fruit, vegetables and wholegrain/multigrain bread and cereal foods. Constipation is managed by ensuring an adequate intake of fibre, an adequate fluid intake and regular physical activity. Soluble fibre supplements are also useful.

Bad breath

Some people choose to limit their carbohydrate intake to help manage their weight. Some find they don't tolerate the carbohydrate-containing foods they did prior to surgery. Whether intentional or not, a diet very low in carbohydrate (less than 100g per day) promotes a state of ketosis. Ketosis occurs when our intake of food, particularly carbohydrate, is low and we burn our fat stores for fuel. This process produces chemicals called ketones. Ketones are removed from the body in our urine but also can be smelled on our breath. Ketosis can also cause dehydration.

Increasing carbohydrate intake will easily treat ketosis and the bad breath that accompanies it. However, it may be that ketosis is an advantage to you at particular times during your journey. Speak to your support team if you are experiencing ketosis.

Hair loss

Healthy human beings are constantly both growing and losing hair, generally growing more than we are losing so we do not notice it. Particular stressors on the body can cause a shift so that we are losing more hair. Two stressors known to do this are major surgery and rapid weight loss. There can also be nutritional causes of hair loss.

Hair loss in the first six months after surgery is generally due to the trauma of the surgery and rapid weight loss. However, with a good nutritional intake it generally settles and hair re-grows as weight loss stabilises.

For hair loss that continues for over a year or starts six months after surgery, particularly in people who have difficulty eating or not taking the supplements recommended to them, there may be a nutritional cause. A low protein intake, iron or zinc deficiency can all play a role in hair loss. However it is important to seek the advice of your team in managing this. It is not appropriate to commence nutritional supplements without guidance, particularly zinc, which when taken in high doses can cause other health concerns.

Lactose intolerance

After gastric bypass surgery, some find they are unable to tolerate as much milk or milk products. It may be that following surgery the body produces less lactase, the enzyme that digests lactose. This may cause temporary or ongoing lactose intolerance. The treatment for this is a low lactose diet or supplementation with the lactase enzyme, which should be discussed with a dietitian. Removing all milk products from the diet is often not necessary and can make you miss out on important nutrients.

Managing hunger

Some people assume that after weight loss surgery they will never be hungry again. It is common for people to have very little appetite in the early stages following gastric bypass or sleeve gastrectomy. Following gastric banding however, it is normal for some people to experience hunger, particularly before the band has been adjusted to find the green zone.

Choosing solid foods rather than liquids and eating regular meals will also help manage your hunger.

Foods high in protein, high in fibre and those with a low glycemic index are generally more satisfying and are great choices to help satisfy you after all types of surgery.

Foods high in protein are discussed elsewhere.

Higher fibre and/or low glycemic index (GI) carbohydrate containing foods should be chosen wherever possible and are also discussed elsewhere.

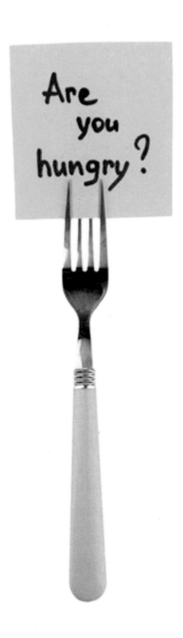

Weight regain

Weight loss surgery is a powerful tool responsible for a significant part of your weight loss. However, it is ultimately your efforts that will prevent you from regaining weight long term. After an initial period of weight loss, weight regain can occur after weight loss surgery and unfortunately weight regain is common. It tends to occur from two years after surgery and it tends to be gradual. Up to 50 percent of people may regain some weight two years or more after surgery. However, whilst most people regain some weight, most are also still classified as 'successful', meaning they maintain a loss of 50 percent or more of their excess body weight.

Maintaining weight loss is challenging. Your body is programmed to have a 'set point' for a weight it prefers. Once you become overweight, your set point will be your maximum weight and your body will try to get back there. Weight loss surgery helps to reset the body's set point, however your body is still, to some extent, always trying to 'defend' its weight.

So often we hear people talk about surgery 'not working' or 'failing'. There are many reasons why surgery may not be successful and it is not simply a matter of the surgery itself 'not working'. A group of experts have examined all the available studies on weight regain following weight loss surgery and come up with five key reasons why people regain weight following surgery. These include:

- Nutritional factors
- Mental health issues
- Hormonal or metabolic causes
- Physical inactivity
- Surgical 'failure'.

We will look at each of these in more detail and then summarise with a checklist that will help you do a quick check of your lifestyle behaviours to either keep you on track, or to help you get back on the path to success.

Nutritional factors

Whilst your energy intake (calories or kilojoules) tends to decrease in the early stages following surgery, over time energy intakes tend to increase and this, not surprisingly, is linked to weight regain. Studies have also found that people who follow the recommended dietary advice early in their weight loss surgery journey are more likely to follow those principles later and tend to lose more weight.

Embracing healthy lifestyle habits is critical for long term weight loss maintenance. Weight regain can occur frighteningly quickly, with one study finding when a person changes their diet, 50 percent of their lost weight can be regained in as little as three months. Poor food choices, poor quality food, grazing and a lack of nutritional guidance and advice are key factors involved in weight gain.

Stay in touch with your dietitian and if your team doesn't have one, seek one out. Find out more about finding a dietitian on page 99. In the meantime, use the checklist at the end of this section to do a quick review of your lifestyle.

Mental health issues

Uncontrolled mental health issues are an important factor in weight regain, including binge eating disorder, depression and other addictive behaviours including alcohol and drug use. There are reports that the more psychiatric conditions a person has, the more weight they will regain.

If you have any mental health concerns that are impacting on your journey, be sure to seek the advice of a psychologist with experience in weight management. If your team does not have their own psychologist, they may be able to refer you to one or you can search for one yourself using the link in the checklist which follows.

Hormonal or metabolic causes

It is possible that following surgery, some people still have imbalances in their hunger hormones that make it challenging to lose weight. It is also possible that reactive hypoglycemia, discussed earlier, interferes with the usual hunger cycle, leading to more regular meals or snacks. Dietary changes can assist in managing this and should be discussed with your dietitian.

Physical inactivity

Studies have shown that people who include moderate or high intensity physical activity tend to lose more weight than those who are not active following weight loss surgery. To continue to lose weight in the long term following surgery, the intensity of physical activity needs to increase. As weight loss generally makes it more comfortable for people to be active, increasing the intensity of activity becomes less challenging than it would have been prior to surgery.

People who do regular physical activity, three to four times per week for at least 30 minutes are less likely to regain their lost weight.

Clearly, a habit of regular physical activity is a key aspect of losing weight and more importantly, maintaining that weight loss long term following weight loss surgery.

Surgical 'failure'

All forms of weight loss surgery carry risks of 'failure'. It can be uncomfortable to use the term 'failure', as it has a negative association. However, many medical treatments need to be revised over time and weight loss surgery is no different.

After gastric band surgery some risk factors for the surgery failing include enlargement of the small pouch above the band, band slippage and reflux. It is possible that any of these complications may cause the band to need to be removed. Following gastric bypass surgery, the small stomach pouch can stretch, as can the stoma, which is the opening from the stomach pouch to the intestine. Both of these factors can make it harder to feel satisfied on a smaller amount of food. The 'sleeve' created following sleeve gastrectomy surgery can also stretch, allowing larger amounts of food to be eaten.

If you are regaining weight the first step is to check that all of the appropriate lifestyle behaviours are in place and the following the checklist can help with this. Whilst all forms of surgery can have complications, a genuine, focused effort on lifestyle change can help turn around what appears to be an unsuccessful surgery. If you are confident that all your lifestyle foundations are in place, you need to raise your concerns with your team. Revisional or 'redo' surgeries are not uncommon and your surgeon would be able to discuss your options with you.

The Weight Regain Checklist

If you are experiencing weight regain, go through this list to identify where you can make changes to get back on track with your weight loss.

Nutritional Issues	Yes	No
Are you still engaged with your dietitian?	O	O
Are you controlling your portion sizes? It can be useful to check your portions – get out your measuring cups, small plates and scales if you need to	O	O
Are you eating beyond the point of feeling satisfied? Try not to see how much you can fit, but rather how little you need to feel satisfied.	O	O
Are you eating too quickly? It can be hard to stop at 'satisfied' if you eat too quickly as you can miss the subtle cues your body gives you. Remember a small meal should take you at least 10 minutes.	O	O
Are you spending too long over meals? Eating over an extended period of time can lead to eating larger portions. As food passes through into your intestine, this leaves room for more. Try not to 'graze' at a meal any longer than 20 minutes.	O	O
Are you drinking with meals? If you have a sleeve gastrectomy or gastric bypass it is important to keep fluids at least 30 minutes away from meal times or it can 'wash' food into your intestine leading to poor satiety and potential over eating.	O	O
Are you consuming adequate protein? It is important to include a minimum of 60g of protein each day to support weight loss (your individual requirements may be higher than this and a dietitian can help you with this). Use an app such as Easy Diet Diary or My Fitness Pal to check how much protein you have each day.	O	O
Are you relying on soft, wet dishes (such as casseroles and stews) and liquid meals? These foods pass through to your intestine faster, therefore are not as satisfying as more solid foods.	O	O
Are you including excess indulgences? Little treats such as chocolate and lollies don't take up much room, but can easily provide excess calories. Take care to limit your intake.	O	O
Are you including at least 1.5L of low energy fluid each day?	O	O
Are you drinking your energy (calories or kilojoules)? Try to limit all high energy fluids such as juice, cordial, sugary hot drinks and alcohol as these are quick to consume, don't leave you satisfied and can make weight loss a challenge.	O	O
Are you grazing? It is so important to avoid grazing following weight loss surgery. Energy quickly adds up in each of those small mouthfuls, but your body doesn't give you the cue to stop. Ensure all food is plated and you sit down to eat.	O	O

Mental Health Issues	Yes	No
Do you experience mental health concerns? Do you have professional support for these concerns? If you don't have a psychologist in your support team to help with your journey, ask your GP whom they would recommend. Alternatively, head to www.psychology.org.au. Go to Find a Psychologist and then search for a psychologist under Weight management.	O	O
Are you eating to manage emotional challenges? Remember, if the problem is not hunger, the answer isn't food. Food only masks the emotion short term. Try to use non food comforts when you are experiencing hard emotional times.	O	O
Are you actively participating in a weight loss surgery support group or network?	O	O
Are you seeking the support of friends and family to help you stay on track?	O	O

Physical Activity	Yes	No
Are you including regular physical activity? Regular meaning three to four times per week, for at least 30 minutes.	O	O
Are you including moderate to high intensity activity?	O	O
Do you need assistance to help formulate a plan to increase your activity? Speak to an Accredited Exercise Physiologist (AEP) to have an exercise program tailored to your needs. An AEP is a university qualified allied health professional. They can provide advice on physical activity and behavioural change for people undergoing weight loss surgery, based on the latest scientific evidence and best practice guidelines for positive outcomes. Find your nearest AEP via Exercise and Sports Science Australia (ESSA): www.aaess.com.au.	O	O

Pregnancy

All women undergoing weight loss surgery should be aware that fertility increases with weight loss. Some women choose to have weight loss surgery to increase their chances of conception, whereas others do not. If you are a woman of reproductive age and not planning a pregnancy, speak to your doctor about contraception following surgery. After gastric bypass surgery, non oral contraceptives are recommended.

Following weight loss surgery, it is important to maximise your nutritional status and manage your body weight to ensure a healthy journey for both you and the baby. It is recommended that you wait 12 to 18 months following weight loss surgery prior to conception.

During pregnancy, your nutrient requirements will increase as the baby grows. Depending on the type of surgery you have had, your ability to obtain nutrients from the foods that you eat may be reduced.

If you find out you are pregnant, planned or not, it is important to inform your support team so they can be involved in your care. They need to request some blood tests or review those you may already have had. Even if you do not have any nutritional deficiencies, monitoring your nutritional status throughout the pregnancy should occur in each trimester. Particular vitamin and mineral supplements may be recommended, different to those you have previously been recommended. For those with a gastric band, this may need adjusting through the course of the pregnancy to enable appropriate weight gain and growth of your baby.

Your support team has the knowledge to guide you through your pregnancy safely, so be sure to utilise them.

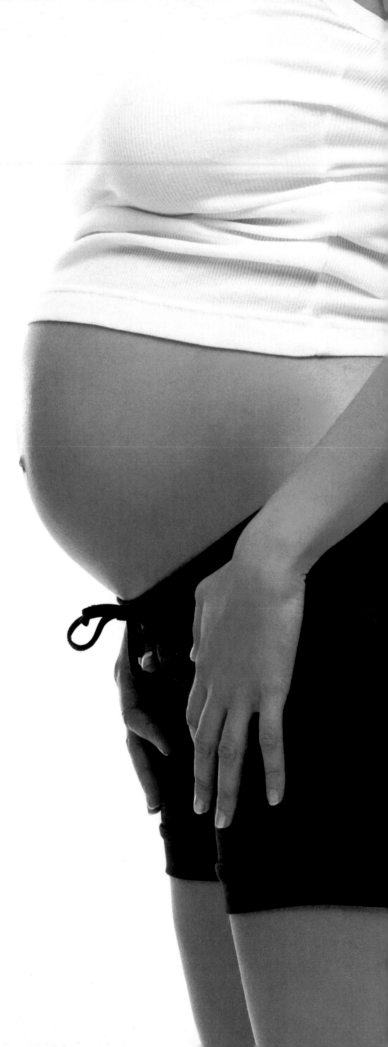

Nutritional Impacts of Weight Loss Surgery and Supplementation

Nutrient Deficiencies

The digestive system remains unchanged after gastric band surgery, hence the risk of nutrient deficiencies is lower than with other surgery types. With a correctly adjusted band you should not experience food intolerances and therefore should be able to eat a balanced diet. However, as you are eating much smaller servings of food you do need to take a multivitamin and mineral supplement to obtain all the nutrients needed for good health.

Gastric bypass surgery changes the anatomy of the digestive system. This means that digestion and absorption of nutrients from food is changed.

As sleeve gastrectomy is a relatively new procedure compared to gastric bypass and gastric band surgeries, there is less information on the nutritional concerns after surgery, however reports of nutrient deficiencies are emerging. For this reason, it is particularly important to return to your surgeon for regular blood tests.

After all forms of weight loss surgery, less food is eaten, hence the risk of nutrient deficiencies increases. The risk of nutrient deficiencies doubles if you do not take the vitamin and mineral supplements recommended to you. An Australian study at the St George Upper GI Clinic found only 40% of people with a gastric band, 70% of people who have had a sleeve gastrectomy and 80% of people who have had a gastric bypass take the vitamin and mineral supplements recommended to them. Health professionals would love these figures to be 100%!

The main nutrients that people may become deficient in following weight loss surgery include:

- protein
- iron
- zinc
- vitamin B12
- thiamin (vitamin B1)
- folate
- vitamin D
- calcium
- fibre.

Following is a description of why we need each of the particular nutrients, where they are found, why you may become deficient following weight loss surgery and preventing deficiencies.

Protein

Why do we need protein?

Protein-containing foods help us feel satisfied for longer after eating, which is helpful in managing our weight.

Protein is also involved in many bodily functions including:

- building and repairing body cells such as bone, hair, skin, nail and muscle
- producing hormones to help us burn stored energy, including body fat
- making enzymes to help digest food
- helping to protect our body against colds, hair loss, muscle weakness, and fatigue.

Not eating enough protein can result in:

- a weaker immune system
- muscle loss
- hair loss
- inadequate weight loss.

Why am I at risk of inadequate protein intake after weight loss surgery?

As indicated in the following protein counter, meat products contain the most protein per serve.

An Australian study from The St George Upper GI Clinic found that those with a gastric band often found red and white meat difficult to tolerate whilst fish was tolerated more easily. Some people who have had sleeve gastrectomy and gastric bypass also reported difficulty eating these foods but it was far less common than it was among those with a gastric band.

Red meat and chicken breast can be more difficult to eat if they are dry, overcooked, stringy, or if they have been reheated. Any meat can be difficult to tolerate if you are not using the correct eating technique. Some people will then avoid these foods,

when working on improving eating technique may allow them to eat these foods comfortably.

Food tolerance varies from person to person and is found by trial and error. Tolerance of all foods can be improved by following the correct eating technique as discussed in the *Food Fundamentals* chapter (page 98) and following the tips to improve food tolerance in the *Troubleshooting and Common Complaints* chapter (page 216).

Following all surgeries, you will be eating smaller amounts of food. A reduced intake of food causes a decrease in protein intake. In the early stages following surgery, people who have had a sleeve gastrectomy or gastric bypass are likely to tolerate only very small quantities of food. When you eat your meals, eat the protein-containing food first to ensure you have room for this important nutrient.

Getting adequate protein

There is no one exact recommended protein intake following weight loss surgery. A minimum intake of 60g has been suggested, however your individual protein needs will vary depending on your age, gender and your particular stage of recovery. It is best to speak to your dietitian about your protein needs. You can then use the protein counter to see how you can achieve this.

Women who are pregnant or breastfeeding need more protein than the general population. If you have had weight loss surgery and are planning a pregnancy, have fallen pregnant or are breastfeeding, you should contact your dietitian, or ask your surgeon to refer you to one.

Monitoring and preventing deficiencies

Albumin, a protein in your blood, is often used as a

way to test if you are deficient in protein. However, this is not the best measure. Prealbumin is a much more effective measure of your nutritional status. This can be ordered on a routine blood test, hence ongoing blood tests are important.

To prevent protein deficiency, ensure a regular intake of protein-containing foods. If you are having difficulty tolerating protein-containing foods, see the *Poor Food Tolerance* section in the *Troubleshooting and Common Complaints* chapter (page 216).

If you would like more detail on the protein content of different foods, protein supplements and bars, check out our Power of Protein book, available via our website: www.nfwls.com.

FOOD	PROTEIN CONTENT PER SERVE
Meat Products	
• 100g cooked (120g raw) meat eg. lean beef, lamb, veal, kangaroo, pork, chicken, fish, mince	25 - 30g
Milk or Milk Products	
• 250ml low fat milk or soy milk • 200g low fat yoghurt • 2 slices (40g) reduced fat cheese • 100g reduced fat ricotta • ¼ cup low fat cottage cheese	9 - 12g
Meat Alternatives	
• 1 egg • 100g cooked tofu • 100g textured vegetable protein (TVP) • ½ cup legumes eg. chick peas, kidney beans, baked beans, three bean mix, broad beans, split peas or lentils • 30g nuts eg. almonds, cashews, etc.	5 - 10g
Breads and Cereals	
• 1 slice bread or fruit bread • ½ cup flaky cereal • 2 Ryvita®crackers	2 - 3g
Vegetables	
• ½ cup cooked vegetables • 1 cup salad vegetables	½ - 3g
Fruits	
• 1 average piece fruit eg. banana, apple, pear, orange	½ - 2g

Iron

Iron is often found in similar foods to protein. The various reasons for a decreased protein intake following surgery have been discussed previously. It is for the same reasons that iron intake often decreases after weight loss surgery.

Why do we need iron?

Iron is essential for healthy blood. It is used by our red blood cells to form haemoglobin, a pigment that carries oxygen to all of our body tissues. Signs that we don't have enough iron in the body include:

- tiredness
- lack of energy
- poor concentration
- frequent infections.

As iron deficiency becomes more severe you can develop brittle nails, a sore mouth, a smooth tongue and painful cracks in the skin at the corners of the mouth.

Why am I at risk of iron deficiency after weight loss surgery?

There is a risk of iron deficiency following all forms of weight loss surgery, with smaller amounts of food being eaten.

Gastric bypass has a greater risk of iron deficiency than other surgeries for two reasons. Firstly, less stomach acid is produced. When we eat foods containing iron, stomach acids convert the iron from a form that is not easily absorbed by the body to a form that is easily absorbed. Secondly, the most efficient area for absorbing iron, the first part of the intestine (the duodenum) is bypassed and food no longer passes through this area. Those who have had gastric bypass surgery should follow the tips to improve iron absorption and include regular iron supplementation. Speak to your surgical team about your iron requirements and supplementation.

Getting adequate iron

Following all forms of weight loss surgery your team should recommend a multivitamin and mineral supplement to you, which should contain iron. Multivitamin and mineral supplements vary enormously in what they contain, so be sure to be advised by a health professional with experience in weight loss surgery and follow their recommendation.

There is no one multivitamin and mineral supplement that is right for everyone after weight loss surgery, just as there is no one amount of iron that is necessary for everyone after surgery. This will depend on your individual blood tests and may vary over time.

After sleeve gastrectomy and gastric bypass surgeries the amount of iron in your diet and a standard multivitamin and mineral supplement is not likely to be adequate. Additional iron supplements will be needed. Some people find iron supplements cause them unpleasant side effects but it is important to not stop taking them without seeking advice. There is a range of supplements of different strength available, so doses can be modified until you find a dose that works for you. Speak with your team about this.

Which foods contain iron?

There are two types of iron in food: Iron from animal foods (called haem iron) and iron from plant foods (called non-haem iron).

The body absorbs haem iron about 10 times better than non-haem iron. Meats are the best source of haem iron. The redder the meat, the higher it is in iron. Therefore beef, lamb and kangaroo are higher in iron than pork, chicken or fish. Fish with coloured flesh such as tuna and mullet, are higher in iron than white fish, such as barramundi.

Non-haem iron is found in some plant foods including wholegrain and iron fortified breads and cereals, legumes, green leafy vegetables, nuts and dried fruit. The table following indicates the iron content of some common foods.

Our body does not absorb non-haem iron as well as haem iron. Including haem iron from animal foods in the same meal will increase the amount of non-haem iron you absorb. You can also increase the iron you absorb from all sources by eating them with foods high in vitamin C, such as fruits and vegetables.

Tea, coffee and unprocessed bran can block the absorption of non-haem iron so should be separated from meals. If you are taking a calcium supplement, it may also bind with iron and prevent it from being absorbed. Iron and calcium supplements should always be taken at opposite ends of the day.

Monitoring and preventing deficiencies

To prevent iron deficiency, ensure a regular intake of iron-containing foods. If you are having difficulty tolerating these foods, particularly red meat, see the *Poor Food Tolerance* section in the *Troubleshooting and Common Complaints* chapter (page 216).

A standard blood test can check your iron levels. If you are found to be iron deficient, this will need to be treated with additional supplements above that recommended to you following surgery and must be discussed with your team.

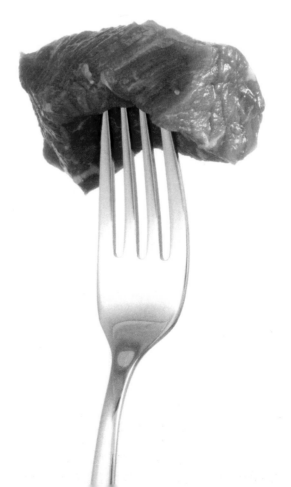

FOOD	IRON CONTENT PER SERVE
Heam Iron Sources	
• 100g cooked liver	9mg
• 120g sardines (one can) • 100g cooked lean beef	3-4mg
• 100g cooked lean lamb	2.5mg
• 100g tuna • 100g cooked lean pork • 1 egg	1-2mg
• 100g cooked fish • 100g cooked lean chicken	<1mg
Non heam Iron Sources	
• ½ cup kidney beans • ½ cup baked beans • ½ cup three bean mix • 2 breakfast biscuits eg. Weetbix®, Vita-brits® • ½ cup cooked spinach • 40g cashews	2-3mg
• 100g tofu • 30g iron fortified breakfast cereal • 10 dried apricot halves	1-2mg
• 1 slice wholemeal/wholegrain/multigrain/white bread • ½ cup cooked mushrooms • 5 prunes • 40g sultanas (small box) • 1 teaspoon Vegemite®	<1mg

Vitamin B12

Why do we need vitamin B12?

Vitamin B12 is involved in:

- making healthy red blood cells
- making nerve cells and providing a protective layer that surrounds nerve cells
- forming our DNA (genetic material)
- metabolism of carbohydrate and fat.

Vitamin B12 has a close relationship with folate, as they depend on each other to work properly.

Vitamin B12 deficiency can result in:

- tiredness and fatigue
- lack of appetite
- depression
- anaemia
- smooth tongue
- breakdown of nerves.

Vitamin B12 deficiency can easily go undetected as symptoms are not always obvious, or symptoms may be blamed on other causes. If B12 deficiency is not detected and continues long term, brain damage can occur. Therefore, regular blood tests to check vitamin B12 is vital.

Why am I at risk of vitamin B12 deficiency after weight loss surgery?

Similar to protein and iron, as meat intake decreases, it is common for B12 intake to decrease.

To absorb vitamin B12 we need stomach acid to release vitamin B12 from protein. We also need intrinsic factor, a protein that helps your intestines absorb vitamin B12, which is produced in the stomach. As gastric band surgery leaves the stomach intact, B12 deficiency is less common. Following sleeve gastrectomy surgery it was thought that less stomach acid and intrinsic factor would be produced. However, little research has been done to indicate this is the case. Surgical teams following those who have had sleeve gastrectomy are not finding an increased rate of B12 deficiency in those who take the supplements recommended to them. Always take the supplements and have the blood tests recommended to you to ensure your B12 levels are within range. After gastric bypass surgery, less stomach acid and intrinsic factor are produced, which, over time, will result in developing a B12 deficiency if not taking the vitamin supplements recommended to you.

Our vitamin B12 stores can last for a year or more after surgery, however keeping these stores relies on not only a regular intake of B12, but also on the ability to absorb it. Only one percent of B12 in supplements will be absorbed. Following gastric bypass surgery, a standard multivitamin and mineral supplement will not provide adequate B12.

Getting adequate vitamin B12

Regular blood tests will indicate whether you are getting adequate vitamin B12 from food and from taking the supplements recommended to you. Some people may find the vitamin B12 in the multivitamin and mineral supplement they are taking adequate to maintain their B12 levels. However, some may need additional supplementation, particularly after gastric bypass surgery.

Vitamin B12 can be taken orally or as injections. If you choose to take a daily supplement, the sublingual forms that dissolve under the tongue are well absorbed. Injections are another effective method of supplementation. For people who have difficulty absorbing vitamin B12, oral tablets are not effective. That is why it is essential to have regular blood tests and speak to your team about your individual needs.

The table following indicates the vitamin B12 content of some common foods. It is important to note that only animal products contain vitamin B12 – it is a myth that mushrooms are a good source of B12!

Monitoring and preventing deficiencies

Vitamin B12 levels can be monitored via blood tests, however a more effective measure is methylmalonic acid (MMA). Early B12 deficiency can be detected if MMA and homocysteine are monitored. It is important for all people to have their B12 status monitored after surgery as obese people generally have a greater risk of B12 deficiency. Make sure you have blood tests at least annually, preferably every six months after gastric bypass and sleeve gastrectomy. If you are not located near your weight loss surgery clinic, arrange this with your GP.

FOOD	VITAMIN B12 CONTENT PER SERVE
• 100g cooked beef liver • 100g cooked lamb kidney	80µg
• 100g oysters • 100g cooked chicken liver	10-20µg
• 100g canned sardines, drained • 100g canned crab, drained	5-10µg
• 100g canned salmon, drained • 100g canned tuna, drained • 100g cooked white fish • 100g cooked lamb • 100g cooked beef • 1 cup low fat milk • 200g low fat yoghurt	1-5µg
• 1 egg • 100g cooked pork • 100g cooked chicken	<1µg

Note: All figures are approximate and sourced from US data on the B12 content of food.

Folate

Why do we need folate?

Folate is a B group vitamin needed for healthy growth and development. It is involved in:

- making enzymes
- making healthy red blood cells
- metabolism of DNA (genetic material)
- preventing neural tube defects in babies during early pregnancy
- reducing homocysteine, an amino acid that can increase our risk of heart disease.

Stores of folic acid in our body can be used up within a few months after surgery unless it is replaced in our diet or from supplements.

Common symptoms in people with folate deficiency include:

- forgetfulness
- irritability
- hostility
- paranoid behaviour.

However, many people will not have any symptoms.

Why am I at risk of folate deficiency after weight loss surgery?

There is a risk of folate deficiency after all forms of weight loss surgery as your intake of folate-containing foods decreases. However, folate deficiency is most likely after gastric bypass as much of the area where folate is absorbed in the intestine is bypassed.

Getting adequate folate

After all forms of weight loss surgery your multivitamin and mineral supplement should contain folate. Having regular blood tests will help determine if you need additional folate. The table following indicates the folate content of some common foods.

Monitoring and preventing deficiencies

A routine blood test can detect if you are low in folate by measuring your level of homocysteine. Homocysteine is an amino acid (a building block of protein) that is produced during a chemical reaction in the body. A high homocysteine level indicates that you may not be getting adequate folate (however it can also indicate vitamin B12 deficiency). Serum and red blood cell folate are also useful to provide more detail on folate deficiency.

FOOD	FOLATE CONTENT PER SERVE
• 100g cooked chicken liver	1400µg
• 100g cooked lamb liver	240µg
• 2 Weetbix® • ½ cup cooked spinach • 5 cooked brussels sprouts • ½ cup cooked broccoli • 5 canned asparagus spears, drained • 5 slices canned beetroot, drained • ½ cup All-Bran® • 1 teaspoon Vegemite®	50-100µg
• ½ cup baked beans	40-50µg
• ½ cup cooked green beans • ½ cup cooked cauliflower/leek/parsnip • 40g cashews • 1 slice wholegrain/multigrain bread • 1 egg	20-40µg
• ½ cup cooked cabbage/carrot • ½ cup mushroom/lettuce • ½ cup strawberries • 40g almonds • 100g cooked beef/chicken/fish • 1 cup low fat milk • 1 medium banana • ½ avocado	Less than 20µg

Zinc

Why do we need zinc?

Zinc plays a role in many bodily functions including:

- wound healing
- our senses of taste, smell and sight
- making of enzymes
- bone strength
- sexual reproduction, particularly in males.

Zinc deficiency can cause:

- poor wound healing
- poor recovery from infections
- skin rashes
- a loss of taste and appetite.

The table following indicates the zinc content of some common foods.

Why am I at risk of zinc deficiency after weight loss surgery?

Red meat is a good source of zinc. If your intake of red meat decreases for reasons described previously, the risk of zinc deficiency increases. Some people may experience diarrhoea after gastric bypass surgery that may be associated with dumping syndrome. As zinc is lost in the faeces, people with diarrhoea are at greater risk of zinc deficiency.

Getting adequate zinc

Zinc should be part of your daily multivitamin and mineral supplement. Doses above this should only be taken if recommended by your support team. High doses of zinc, when taken without supervision, can cause other health concerns.

Monitoring and preventing deficiencies

Taking zinc as part of your daily multivitamin and mineral supplement should prevent zinc deficiency in most people. If you have long-term diarrhoea after gastric bypass surgery, discuss with your support team.

FOOD	ZINC CONTENT PER SERVE
• 100g oysters	65mg
• 100g cooked lean beef • 100g cooked lean lamb • 100g cooked lean beef mince	5mg
• 100g cooked lean pork • 100g cooked lean chicken	1-5mg
• 100g cooked fish • 1 egg	<1mg

Thiamin (Vitamin B1)

Why do we need thiamin?

Thiamin helps to convert glucose into energy, plays a role in normal appetite and digestion and has a role in proper functioning of our heart and nervous system.

Symptoms of thiamin deficiency include confusion and irritability, poor arm and/or leg coordination, lethargy, fatigue and muscle weakness.

Why am I at risk of thiamin deficiency after weight loss surgery?

Thiamin deficiency can occur after all forms of weight loss surgery. Without a regular, adequate intake of thiamin our body stores can quickly run out. Regular vomiting can also deplete thiamin stores in a short time.

Thiamin deficiency is more likely after gastric bypass as thiamin is absorbed in the areas of the intestine that are bypassed during surgery.

Getting adequate thiamin

After all surgeries, thiamin should be part of the daily multivitamin and mineral supplement. If you have ongoing nausea and/or vomiting following surgery, you may require additional thiamine supplements and should discuss this with your support team. If thiamin deficiency goes undetected, you can develop short-term memory loss and irreversible nerve/muscle disorders.

The table following indicates the thiamin content of some common foods.

Monitoring and preventing deficiencies

If you are experiencing persistent vomiting after any form of weight loss surgery, you are at risk of thiamin deficiency as well as more serious irreversible complications. Please contact your support team as soon as possible to arrange tests.

FOOD	THIAMIN CONTENT PER SERVE
• 1 teaspoon Vegemite® • 1 teaspoon Marmite®	1mg
• ½ cup peanuts • 100g cooked lean pork	0.5 – 0.9mg
• ½ cup cashews/pistachios • ½ cup All-Bran® • 1 Weetbix®	0.3 – 0.5mg
• ½ cup walnuts/almonds • 100g cooked kidney/liver • 1 tablespoon sesame seeds • 1 slice wholemeal/grain bread • 1 potato • ½ cup cooked peas/broad beans/kidney beans • ½ cup bran flakes	0.1 – 0.2mg

Calcium and Vitamin D

Why do we need calcium and vitamin D?

Calcium is a mineral that helps to build and maintain healthy bones. It is also involved in blood clotting, nerve and muscle function. When the calcium level in the blood falls too low and we are not getting enough from our diet, our body draws calcium out of the bones. A diet low in calcium means we are constantly drawing on the bones, decreasing bone strength. If this continues long term it can result in osteoporosis.

Vitamin D helps the body absorb calcium and a Vitamin D deficiency can increase the risk of developing osteoporosis. The body produces vitamin D naturally when skin is exposed to sunlight during everyday activities.

Why am I at risk of calcium and vitamin D deficiency after weight loss surgery?

All people are at risk of low vitamin D levels if they do not get enough sun exposure. Being obese is a further risk factor for vitamin D deficiency. A study at the St George Upper GI Clinic in Sydney found approximately 60% of people coming to them prior to having surgery had a vitamin D deficiency.

A low calcium intake from a reduced dietary intake and/or not taking the recommended supplements can occur after all forms of surgery. Gastric bypass surgery bypasses some parts of the intestine where calcium is absorbed, making it harder for the body to absorb enough calcium. Those having gastric bypass surgery are therefore at the greatest risk of bone disorders following surgery.

Getting adequate calcium and vitamin D

After weight loss surgery 1200 to 1500 mg of calcium per day is recommended. The following table indicates the calcium content of some common foods. Many people will need calcium supplements in addition to the calcium they obtain from food. There are particular types of calcium supplements that are recommended, as they are better absorbed, particularly after gastric bypass and sleeve gastrectomy surgeries.

An Australian position paper details the level of sun exposure that is likely to help maintain adequate vitamin D levels in the body. It is recommended that for moderately fair-skinned people, a walk with arms exposed for six to seven minutes mid morning or mid afternoon in summer should be adequate. In winter, that walk should be with as much bare skin exposed as possible, for seven to 40 minutes (depending on latitude) around noon. This should occur on most days. When sun exposure is limited, supplementation is likely to be required. This should be assessed on an individual basis.

Monitoring and preventing deficiencies

A blood test will indicate the level of calcium in the blood, but not in the bones. Unfortunately the level of calcium in the blood will not decrease until osteoporosis has severely depleted the stored calcium in the bones.

A blood test will measure Vitamin D levels. Vitamin D deficiency is common in obese people. Those who are vitamin D deficient will need a high replacement dose/s of vitamin D. Different clinics will have different protocols for managing this. Discuss with your support team.

FOOD	CALCIUM CONTENT PER SERVE
<ul><li>1 cup (250ml) low fat, reduced fat or soy milk</li><li>200g low fat yoghurt</li><li>2 slices cheese</li><li>½ cup ricotta cheese</li><li>½ cup canned salmon, drained (with bones)</li></ul>	300mg

Fibre

Why do we need fibre?

A high fibre diet:

- helps prevent constipation
- improves weight control by helping to make us feel satisfied
- improves diabetes management by helping to slow the absorption of glucose into the blood
- decreases the risk of heart disease as soluble fibres can help remove cholesterol from the body
- helps protect against bowel cancer, haemorrhoids, irritable bowel syndrome and diverticulitis.

There are two types of fibre and both are important for good health:

1. **Soluble fibre** forms a gel-like solution and slows down stomach emptying, digestion and absorption of food. Soluble fibre is found in oats, barley, lentils, peas, seed husks, psyllium, some fruits and vegetables.
2. **Insoluble fibre** absorbs water in the large intestine, making our stools softer and bulkier. Insoluble fibre is found in cereals, the skins of fruits and vegetables, nuts, seeds, wholegrain foods.

Why am I at risk of getting inadequate fibre after weight loss surgery?

When eating smaller amounts of food after weight loss surgery, your intake of fibrous foods such as fresh fruits and vegetables, salads and wholegrain/multigrain breads will generally decrease. As you are limited in the quantities you can eat, choose the high fibre options wherever possible such as brown rice, wholemeal pasta and wholegrain/multigrain breads and cereals.

How much fibre do I need?

There is no specific recommendation for fibre intake for those who have had weight loss surgery. The best available guideline is the Australian Nutrient Reference Values that recommends 25-30g of fibre per day.

The table following indicates the fibre content of some common foods.

Monitoring and preventing deficiencies

Try to always choose the higher fibre varieties when choosing bread, cereal, rice and pasta. Include fruits and vegetables with skins wherever possible and be sure to chew them well. Include legumes in salads, casseroles or stews regularly.

If additional fibre is needed, Benefiber® can be added to fluids and some foods. It is colourless, tasteless and doesn't thicken like some fibre supplements, so can easily be added to a range of foods to boost your fibre intake.

FOOD	FIBRE CONTENT PER SERVE
• ½ cup All-Bran®	10g
• ½ cup natural muesli • ½ cup canned, drained beans including kidney beans/baked beans/three bean mix • ½ cup cooked spinach/peas • 1 tablespoon psyllium husk (only use when fully recovered from surgery as this can swell in the stomach).	5 – 7g
• 40g almonds/peanuts/pistachios • ½ cup bran flakes/Sultana Bran®/Just Right® • ½ cup cooked wholemeal pasta • 1 apple/pear • ½ cup cooked broad beans/chick peas • ½ cup cooked broccoli • Benefiber® (2 teaspoons provides 3g fibre)	3 – 4g
• 40g walnuts/cashews • ½ cup cooked corn/carrot/pumpkin • 1 cooked potato • ½ cup Sustain® • 1 orange/banana	2 – 3g
• 1 Weetbix®/Vita-brits® • ½ cup cooked porridge • ½ cup cooked brown rice • ½ cup cooked white pasta • 1 slice wholemeal/grain bread • 1 slice fruit loaf • 1 Ryvita®/Vita-weat®/wholemeal Salada®/wholemeal premium • 1 tablespoon pumpkin/sesame seeds • 1 apricot • ½ cup cooked cauliflower/green beans	1 – 2g
• ½ cup Special K®/puffed wheat/cornflakes/Rice Bubbles®/Nutri-grain® • ½ cup cooked white rice • 1 slice white bread • 1 Cruskits®/Salada®/Sao®	<1g

Supplementation Summary

Vitamin and mineral supplementation following weight loss surgery is highly individual. It depends on your individual health status and the form of surgery you have had. You should always be guided by the health professionals in your weight loss surgery team. Regular blood tests will ensure your team can recommend the best supplements for you.

It is important to take the vitamin and mineral supplements recommended to you not only to prevent nutrient deficiencies that can occur following weight loss surgery, but also to enhance weight loss and prevent weight regain.

You must include the vitamin and mineral supplements recommended to you for life. Simply feeling good or having more energy does not mean that you have a nutritionally adequate diet and are free from nutrient deficiencies.

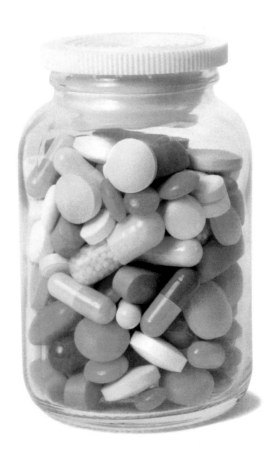

References

- ACOG Practice Bulletin: Bariatric Surgery and Pregnancy, Obstetrics and Gynecology. 2009: 113(6).
- Aills L, Blankenship MS, Buffington C et al. ASMBS Allied Health Nutritional Guidelines for the Surgical Weight Loss Patient. Surgery for Obesity and Related Diseases 2008; 4:S73-S108.
- Apovian CM, Cummings S, Anderson W et al. Best Practice Updates for Multidisciplinary Care in Weight Loss Surgery. Obesity 2009; 17(5):871-879.
- Australian Government, Department of Health and Ageing, National Health & Medical Research Council. Nutrient reference values for Australian and New Zealand, including recommended dietary intakes. Commonwealth of Australia, 2006.
- Avinoah E, Ovnat A and Charuzi I. Nutritional status seven years after Roux-en-Y gastric bypass surgery. Surgery 1992; 111(2):137-42.
- Bauzon, Helen. www.helenbauzon.com
- Behrns K, Smith C, Sarr M. Prospective evaluation of gastric acid secretion and cobalamin absorption following gastric bypass for clinically severe obesity. Digestive Diseases and Sciences 1994; 39(2):315–320.
- Brolin RE. Weight gain after short- and long-limb gastric bypass in patients followed for longer than 10 years. Annals of Surgery 2007; 246(1):163–4; author reply 164.
- Brolin RE, Gorman JH, Gorman RC et al. Prophylactic iron supplementation after Roux-en-Y gastric bypass: A prospective, double blind, randomized study. Archives of Surgery 1998; 133(7):740-4.
- Brown WA, Burton PR, Anderson M et al. Symmetrical Pouch Dilatation After Laparoscopic Adjustable Gastric Banding: Incidence and Management. Obesity Surgery 2008; 18:1104-1108.
- Burton PR, Yap K, Brown WA et al. Changes in Satiety, Supra- and Infraband Transit, and Gastric Emptying Following Laparoscopic Adjustable Gastric Banding: A Prospective Follow-up Study. Obesity Surgery 2011; 21(2):217-223.
- Carswell K, Vincent R, Belgaumkar A et al. The Effect of Bariatric Surgery on Intestinal Absorption and Transit Time. Obesity Surgery 2014; 24(5): 796-805.
- Chevallier JM, Paita M, Rodde-Dunet MH et al. Predictive Factors of Outcome After Gastric Banding: A Nationwide Survey on the Role of Center Activity and Patients' Behaviour. Annals of Surgery 2007; 246(6):1034-1039.
- Clark A. (2012). Portion Perfection for Bands and Sleeves: Seeing is understanding. Great Ideas in Nutrition.
- Colles SL, Dixon JB, O'Brien PE. Hunger Control and Regular Physical Activity Facilitate Weight Loss After Laparoscopic Adjustable Gastric Banding. Obesity Surgery 2008; 18: 833-840.
- Colles S, Dixon J, Marks P et al. Preoperative weight loss with a very-low-energy diet: quantitation of changes in liver and abdominal fat by serial imaging. Am J Clin Nutr 2006; 84:304 –11.
- Compher CW, Hanlon A, Kang Y et al. Attendance at Clinical Visits Predicts Weight Loss After Gastric Bypass Surgery. Obesity Surgery 2012; 22(6):927-934.
- Cook CM, Edwards C. Success Habits of Long-Term Gastric Bypass Patients. Obesity Surgery 1999; 9:80-82.
- Dietitians Association of Australia. Best practice guidelines for the treatment of overweight & obesity in adults [internet]. Australia: Dietitians Association of Australia. Available from: http://dmsweb.daa.asn.au/dmsweb/frmDINERDetails.aspx?id=75

- Dixon JB, O'Brien PE. Nutritional Outcomes of Bariatric Surgery. In: Buchwald H, Cowen G, ed. Bariatric Surgery: WB Saunders 2003; 3-13.

- Dixon J, Reuben Y, Halket, C et al. Shoulder Pain is a Common Problem Following Laparoscopic Adjustable Gastric Band Surgery. Obesity Surgery 2005; 15:1111-1117.

- Dixon JB, Strauss BJG, Laurie C et al. Changes in body composition with weight loss: obese subjects randomized to surgical and medical programs. Obesity 2007; 15(5):1187-1198.

- Faria SL, Kelly EDO, Linz RD et al. Nutritional Management of Weight Regain After Bariatric Surgery 2010; 20(2):135-139.

- Flanagan L. Measurement of Functional Pouch Volume following Gastric Bypass Procedure. Obesity Surgery 1996; 6:38-43.

- Guisti V, Suter M, Heraief E et al. Effects of Laparoscopic Gastric Banding on Body Composition, Metabolic Profile and Nutritional Status of Obese Women: 12-Months Follow-Up. Obesity Surgery 2004: 14:239-245.

- Hamdy O, Snow K, Srinivasan V. Hypoglycemia Clinical Presentation [internet] Available from: http://emedicine.medscape.com/article/122122-clinical. Accessed 23/6/16.

- Heart Foundation http://heartfoundation.org.au/news/eat-fish-for-a-healthy-heart Accessed 25/6/16.

- Hill JO, Sparling PB, Shields TW et al. Effects of exercise and food restriction on body compostion and metabolic rate in obese women. American Journal of Clinical Nutrition, 1987; 46:622-30.

- Jacques J. The latest on nutrition and hair loss in the bariatric patient. Available: http://bariatrictimes.com/the-latest-on-nutrition-and-hair-loss-in-the-bariatric-patient/ Accessed 9/1/2014.

- Jammah AA. Endocrine and metabolic complications after bariatric surgery. Saudi J Gastroenterol 2015; 21:269-77.

- Jarman C, Cohen L. Gastric Volume Trial - A 5 year Update. Obesity Surgery Society Australia and New Zealand Conference, April 2012.

- Jones L, Jones K, Bertuch R et al. Solid versus liquid – satiety study in well adjusted lap-band patients. Obesity Surgery Society Australia and New Zealand Conference, April 2012.

- Karlsson J, Taft C, Ryden A et al. Ten-year trends in health-related quality of life after surgical and conventional treatment for severe obesity: the SOS intervention study. International Journal of Obesity 2007; 31(8):1248-61.

- Karmali S, Brar B, Shi X et al. Weight recidivism post-bariatric surgery: a systematic review. Obesity Surgery 2013; 23(11):1922-33.

- Keren D, Matter I, Rainis T et al. Getting the Most from the Sleeve: The Importance of Post-Operative Follow-up. Obesity Surgery 2011; 12:1887-1893.

- Kruseman M, Leimgruber A, Zumback F, Golay A. Dietary, Weight, and Psychological Changes among Patients with Obesity, 8 Years after Gastric Bypass. Journal of the American Dietetic Association 2010; 110:527-534.

- Love AI, Billett HH. Obesity, bariatric surgery, and iron deficiency: True, true, true and related. American Journal of Hematology 2008; 83(5):403-9.

- Magro DO, Geloneze B, Delfini R et al. Long-term weight regain after gastric bypass: a 5-year prospective study. Obesity Surgery 2008; 18:648–51.

- McMahon MM, Sarr MG, Clark MM et al. Clinical Management After Bariatric Surgery: Value of a

Multidisciplinary Approach. Mayo Clin Proc 2006; 81:S34-S45.

- Mechanick J, Kushner R, Sugerman H et al. ASMBS Guidelines. American Association of Clinical Endocrinologists, The Obesity Society, and American Society for Metabolic & Bariatric Surgery Medical Guidelines for Clinical Practice for the Perioperative Nutritional, Metabolic, and Nonsurgical Support of the Bariatric Surgery Patient. Surgery for Obesity and Related Diseases 2008; 4:S109-S184.

- Mechanick J, Youdin A, Jones D et al. Clinical Practice Guidelines for the Perioperative Nutritional, Metabolic, and Nonsurgical Support of the Bariatric Surgery Patient – 2013 Update: Cosponsored by American Association of Clinical Endocrinologists, The Obesity Society, and American Society for Metabolic & Bariatric Surgery. Endocrine Practice 2013; 19(2):337-72.

- Moize VL, Pi-Sunyer X, Mochari H et al. Nutritional Pyramid for Post-gastric Bypass Patients. Obesity Surgery 2010; 20:1133-1141.

- Optifast VLCD Clinical Treatment Protocol. Available: http://www.optifast.com.au/~/media/487E23A2542 D40B7A9736B7577F88AB0.ashx. Accessed 25/6/16.

- NHMRC Alcohol Guidelines. Available: https://www.nhmrc.gov.au/health-topics/alcohol-guidelines. Accessed 25/6/16.

- Novais PFS, Rassera I, Shiragw EC et al. Food Aversions in Women During The 2 Years After Roux-En-Y Gastric Bypass. Obesity Surgery 2011; 21:1921-1927

- Nowson CA, McGrath JJ, Ebeling PR et al. Vitamin D and health in adults in Australia and New Zealand: a position statement. Medical Journal of Australia 2012; 196(11):686-687.

- O'Brien PE. Gastric Banding and the Fine Art of Eating. Available: http://bariatrictimes.com/gastric-banding-and-the-fine-art-of-eating/comment-page-1/ Accessed 25/6/16.

- Olsen, RH, Krogh-Madsen R, Thomsen C et al. Metabolic Responses to Reduced Daily Steps in Healthy Nonexercising Men, Journal of the American Medical Association 2008; 299(11):1261-1263.

- Overs SE, Freeman RA, Zarshenas N et al. Food Tolerance and Gastrointestinal Quality of Life Following Three Bariatric Procedures: Adjustable Gastric Banding, Roux-en-Y Gastric Bypass, and Sleeve Gastrectomy 2012; 22:536-543.

- Palazuelos-Genis T, Mosti M, Sanchez-Leenheer S et al. Weight Loss and Body Composition During the First Postoperative Year of a Laparoscopic Roux-En-Y Gastric Bypass. Obesity Surgery 2008; 18:1-4.

- Parkes E. Nutritional Management of Patients after Bariatric Surgery. American Journal of Medical Sciences 2006; 331(4):207-213.

- Pritchard J. Review of Protein requirements During Weight Loss. Personal Communication 2011.

- Royal Australasian College of Surgeons and The Obesity Surgery Society of Australia & New Zealand. Weight Loss Surgery. A guide for patients about bariatric surgery. Edition 1, May 2009.

- Shah M, Simha V, Garg A. Review: long-term impact of bariatric surgery on body weight, comorbidities and nutritional status. The Journal of Clinical Endocrinology and Metabolism 2006; 91:4223–31.

- Singh E, Vella A. Hypoglycemia After Gastric Bypass Surgery. Diabetes Spectrum 2012; 25(4): 217-21.

- Snyder-Marlow G, Taylor D, Lenhard MJ. Nutrition Care for Patients Undergoing Laparoscopic Sleeve Gastrectomy for Weight Loss. Journal of the American Dietetic Association 2010; 110:600-607.

- Steigler P, Cunliffe A. The Role of Diet and Exercise for the Maintenance of Fat-Free Mass and Resting Metabolic Rate During Weight Loss. Sports Medicine 2006; 36(3):239-262.

- The University of Sydney. Glycemic Index Database [intenet]. Available from: www.glycemicindex.com/

foodSearch.php Accessed 9/7/12.

- Thomas JR, Gizis F, Marcus E. Food Selections of Roux-en-Y Gastric Bypass Patients up to 2.5 Years Postsurgery. Journal of the American Dietetic Association 2010; 110:608-612.

- Toh SY, Zarshenas N, Jorgensen J. Prevalence of nutrient deficiencies in bariatric patients. Nutrition 2009; 25(11):1150-1156.

- Tzovaras G, Papamargaritis D, Sioka E, et al. Symptoms suggestive of dumping syndrome after provocation in patients after laparoscopic sleeve gastrectomy. Obesity Surgery 2012; 22(1):23-8.

- Ukleja A. 2006. Dumping Syndrome. Practical Gastroenterology; Feb 2006:32-46.

- Williams T. Comparative nutrient review of products formulated or promoted for weight loss by life stage, gender and body weight. Obesity Surgery Society Australia and New Zealand Conference, April 2012.

- Zarshenas N. Nutritional management in gastric bypass and sleeve gastrectomy. Personal communication May 2011.

Index

At Nutrition for Weight Loss Surgery
we offer a whole range
of weight loss surgery specific
tools, products and support options.

Be sure to check us out at
www.nfwls.com